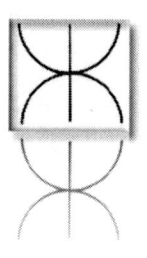

The Sphere of Art II

Aesch Mezareph

The Purifying Fire

Spiritual Alchemy and New Qabalah
for the 21st Century

By
R. J Stewart

R. J. Stewart Books

The Sphere of Art II : Aesch Mezareph
The Purifying Fire, Spiritual Alchemy and New Qabalah
for the 21st Century.
By R. J. Stewart

Published by R. J. Stewart Books
PO Box 58 Dexter, OR 97431

All rights reserved under the Pan-American and International Copyright Conventions. This book may not be reproduced in whole or in part in any form or by any means electronic or mechanical including photocopying recording or by any information storage and retrieval system, include the Internet, now known or hereinafter invented without written permission from the publisher. Contact: www.rjstewart.net

Cover art © Jerry Gehringer 2012

The moral right of the author has been asserted.
Copyright 2012 © First edition
Printed in the United State of America

A catalogue record for this book is available from the Library of Congress.

ISBN: 978-09819246-9-4

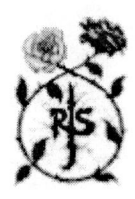

An Inner Temple Traditions/Inner Convocation ® Publication

Biography

R.J. Stewart is a Scottish author, musician, and composer of international acclaim, who has composed for theater, film, and television, toured as a concert performer, and has made many recordings of his own music. He lives in a remote part of Northern California. He has researched and written extensively on the spiritual and sacromagical core of the Western esoteric traditions, with forty-three books in publication translated into many languages worldwide.

R.J. Stewart works with myth, imagination, music and the primal magical arts of vision and inner transformation. Since 1989 he has concentrated mainly on writing and on teaching small groups in Britain and the USA, working toward the regeneration of esoteric traditions for practical contemporary use.

The Sphere of Art (Volumes One and Two) contains the most advanced techniques taught and practiced within the Inner Temple Traditions/Inner Convocation ® program created and presented internationally by the author from its inception in 1989 to the present day.

Acknowledgements

I wish to acknowledge the profound spiritual influence of Alfred Ronald Heaver through personal meetings in the 1970's, the dynamic teaching of William Gordon Gray and Roberta Gray in the same decade, the perceptive spiritual advice of Kathleen Raine, and the support of Gareth Knight. Special thanks to my partner Anastacia Nutt for reading, commenting on, and editing the original manuscript, and for creating many of the illustrations. As always, a substantial thanks is owed to the students and friends worldwide who have worked with the author in opening the *Sphere of Art* as a sacromagical and theurgic path for the 21st century. The cover art was painted by Jerry Gehringer, from his visionary experiences within the *Sphere of Art* .

CONTENTS

How to Read and Use this Book 6
Preface 11
Introduction 17
Chapter One: Theurgy, Thaumaturgy, High and Low Magic 23
Chapter Two: Planetary Forces, Working to Scale 45
Chapter Three: Elevating the Seven Metals 71
Chapter Four: The Four Holy Fires 95
Chapter Five: The Tree of Life, the Sphere of Art 107
Chapter Six: Chaos Eros and Cosmos 127
Chapter Seven: *Aesch Mezareph*: Elucidation 141
Appendix One: Preparing and Diluting from a Matrix 176
Appendix Two: Working with Inner Contacts 178
Appendix Three: The Sphere of Art (from the audio CD) 189
Appendix Four: Expanding Sequence of Angels 194
Appendix Five: Paths, Metals, and Tarot Trumps 202
Appendix Six: Preface to 19th century edition
of *Aesch Mezareph*, by Dr W. Wynn Westcott 204
Appendix Seven: *Aesch Mezareph,* Chapter One,
18th century edition, by "A Lover of Philalethes" (1714) 207
Notes and Reference Sources 245

ILLUSTRATIONS : PAGE 211-243

Figure One: The Tree of Life
Figure Two: The Three Worlds of Moon Sun and Stars
Figure Three: Seven Planets Enfolding
Figure Four: Sevenfold Directions
Figure Five: Interaction of Force and Form
Figure Six: The Rising Earth Light
Figure Seven: Archangels upon the Tree of Life

Figure Eight: The Three Wheels
Figure Nine: The Three Vessels
Figure Ten: The Triplicities
Figure Eleven: The Wheel of Life
Figure Twelve: The Pattern of Ten Vials
Figure Thirteen: Connections Above and Below
Figure Fourteen: The Four Holy Fires
Figure Fifteen: The OverWorld and UnderWorld Tree
Figure Sixteen: Chaos, Cosmos, and Eros
Figure Seventeen: Triads of the Tree, Threefold Alliances
Figure Eighteen: The Long Triads of the Tree
Figure Nineteen: The Solar Emanations
Figure Twenty: The Nested Emanations
Figure Twenty One: The Numeric Progression of Angels
Figure Twenty Two: Sigils of the Archangels
Figure Twenty Three: Archangels and Angels on the Tree
Figure Twenty Four: Turning About the Wheel
Figure Twenty Five: OverWorld - UnderWorld
Figure Twenty Six: Hexagram and Pentagram
Figure Twenty Seven: The Supernal Triad
Figure Twenty Eight: The Tree as Nested Spheres
Figure Twenty Nine: Elemental Tree of Life
Figure Thirty: Reconciling the Worlds
Figure Thirty One: The Multifold Tree of Life (1973)
Figure Thirty Two: The Threefold Tree of Life (1978)

The sages use not violent flames nor burning coals like the vulgar Chemists but imitate Nature and work with her fire: a fire vaporous and yet not light, a fire which nourishes and devours not, a fire natural and yet made by art, dry yet causing rain, moist and yet drying, a water which quenches, a water which washes the body and yet moistens not the hands.

(From Sir Isaac Newton's hand-written translation of
La Lumiere sortant des Tenebres c. 1687-1692)

How To Read and Use This Book

This book combines theory and practice. Or perhaps not, because there is no such thing as "theory" in esoteric tradition, only a series of dissolving maps that lead to changes of perception. So we might instead say this book combines indicators toward transformative spiritual practice. *Four essential parts* first explore such indicators, describing their origins, and how they might be used; next come *two intensely practical parts*; then *three further explorations* and expositions. The reader may be inspired to jump directly to the practical parts, and who am I to say "no, you must rein yourself in"? I will say it anyway, for without studying the preceding indicators for practice, and then studying the subsequent explorations and conceptual discussions, the practical work may seem impractical and more difficult than it truly is.

As always with books on esoteric subjects, it is best to first read steadily through from cover to cover, chapter by chapter, as if reading a novel. This helps to seat the practices and their supporting indicators into the imagination. I recommend doing this without making notes, and while in a gentle meditative state, without interruption from communications or media in any form. *Turn them all off.*

Next read the book again carefully from the beginning, making as many notes as you like, and when you come to the practical chapters, commence your work! Read the remaining chapters and appendices, making whatever notes inspire you, while you are resting between your sacromagical and theurgic labors, during the periods between each phase of your practical work. The plan of the book is thus:

The first four parts: *Preface, Introduction*, and *Chapters One* and *Two* contain essential indicators and concepts, definitions of vocabulary, and many clarifications of ideas and terms that are often deeply embedded in unquestioned usage.

The practical program: *Chapters Three* and *Four* contain a detailed set of practical exercises or *forms*; there are also many other indicators for meditation scattered throughout the book.

The four subsequent parts: *Chapters Five* and *Six* return to exploring indicators, in detail, for spiritual practice with *Aesch Mezareph, Purifying Fire*, and the *Sphere of Art*. *Chapter Seven* is a short elucidation of the first part of the original text, *Aesch Mezareph*, which contains many insights from the historic text.

The seven short Appendices: 1,2,3,4, and 5 are essential supplements to the practical work, and should be studied carefully; 6 and 7 are reference items, for historical interest.

The topics in each Chapter are as follows:

PREFACE, 11

The Efflorescent Tree/How much can be taught through text?/The Scrambled Order/The New Way/What is left out?

INTRODUCTION, 17

The three sources of Aesch Mezareph in this book: The historic text/ The mystical phrase/ The quiet gravestone.

CHAPTER ONE, 23

Theurgy and Thaumaturgy: High and Low Magic/Inside the Activated Sphere of Art/The sacromagical process of redemption and evolution/Alchemy and Evolution.

Beyond Dualism: The Threefold Interaction/What is given back? /The Redemption of Energy /What did we lose, and who gives it back? /The Map and the Territory/The Tree of Life replaces the Map/The enfolding and interleaved territories.

Explanations of spiritual awareness and transformation: Dissolving Map, Redeeming Mind/The Childhood Explorer.

Pins on the Map: The Inner Temples/ Inner-Plane Contacts.

CHAPTER TWO, 45

Working to Scale: Telluric and Stellar Realities/The problem of pseudo-knowledge

Forgetting where we are: We exist within and through the Seven Directions/ Invocation Evocation and Power/Energy, Form, and Consciousness.

The interaction point: Riding the Chariot, Uplifting the World/The Four Guardians or Archangels/Planetary Intelligences defined/The Significance and Function of the Four Archangels or Guardians/UnderWorld Considerations.

The Archangels and the Metals: The Four Archangels in sequence, from Earth to Sun/Archangels and Gender: The Gender Meditation/The Archangelic Cycle of the Elements/Telesms of power in action/Archangels as Mirrors and Lenses. The Three Vessels.

CHAPTER THREE, 71

Working with the Metals:/The Dry Way and the Wet Way/The Metals and Substances defined/ Sulfur, Salt, and Mercury/The Elemental Cycle of Transformation.

Practical Work (1): The Dry materials, A Period of Rest

Practical Work (2): The Wet Materials

Conclusion: The Dry Way, the Wet Way, the Elevation

CHAPTER FOUR, 95

The Four Holy Fires: Moving the Four Holy Fires through the Elements within the Body/Rising from the UnderWorld/the Combustion Cycle/The Primary Affinities/The Secondary Affinities.

Summary of Sphere of Art Practices utilizing Aesch Mezareph, The Cord and the Sphere.

CHAPTER FIVE, 107

Emanations of the Tree of Life within the Sphere of Art: Elucidation of the Sphere of Art/Teaching and Transmission.

The Physical Space: The Temple Not Built With Hands/Sacred Geometry/Threefold Interaction within the Physical Space/

Working with the Three Zones/The Platonic Solids/Shapes and Energies within a Sphere.

Creating the Cosmos: Less is always More/Using the Tree of Life, or not? / What Tree of Life may be aligned within the Sphere of Art? / Words of Caution and of Liberation/the OverWorld and UnderWorld Trees/The Evolution of Metals/Energizing and Emptying the Sphere.

CHAPTER SIX, 127

Chaos Eros and Cosmos: In the Beginning/The Laws of Magic and the Sphere of Art/If there are hidden laws, what are they hiding from? /Undo what you will/Is Chaos untidy?

To counter the threat of nuclear Armageddon: Evil as Energy/Compassion and Coercion.

CHAPTER SEVEN, 141

An elucidation of the first chapter of Aesch-Mezareph, the Purifying Fire: Preamble/ Kabbalistic Origins/ The Translations of Aesch Mezareph/Humor and Hyper-text/The Original Plan/the Eight Chapters Unfold/Depths of Allusion...or Illusion?

The Original Text quoted and examined: Elisha and the Fire Temple Tradition/The Supernal Triad emerging from the Void/The Sevenfold Immersion/Ethics, Needs, and Wants/The River of Judgment/The Descending and Ascending Rivers/Changing Direction.

The Emanations and the Metals are at One: Intentional Confusion provokes thought/Correcting the Metals/The White and Red Natures/The Solar Emanations, Lesser Countenance, and *Shekinah*/Uplifting the Lunar Triad/The Two Faces, or Long Triads of the Stellar and Solar Realms/The Lunar Realm and Living Water.

Coming to Earth: The Three Supernal Emanations as allegorical Sulphur, Salt, and Mercury/The Seven Lower Emanations as the Seven Metals/Balancing the Kings of Edom/Mysteries of the *Shekinah* and the Ark. *Conclusion.*

APPENDIX ONE, 176 : *Preparing and Diluting from a Matrix.*

APPENDIX TWO, 178: *Working with Inner Contacts:* The nuts and bolts of spiritual communication/The basic information/Some classic cautions/Beware of Stereotypes/The Neighborhood Analogy/The Positive and Beneficial aspects/All Things Reversed.

APPENDIX THREE, 189 : *The Sphere of Art,* audio script, from the audio CD "The Sphere of Art": Introduction/Building the Sphere of Art/The Sanctuary of Avalon Vision.

APPENDIX FOUR, 194: *Expanding Sequence of Angels:* The flow and return of the Emanations/The Reconciliation of the Worlds/The Emanations of the Tree of Life/Orders of Archangels and their Angels/Crossing the Bridge/toward the Sacred Earth.

APPENDIX FIVE, 202: *Paths, Metals, and Tarot Trumps*

APPENDIX SIX, 204: Preface to 19th century edition of Aesch Mezareph, by Dr. W. Wynn Westcott.

APPENDIX SEVEN, 207: *Aesch Mezareph,* Chapter One, 18th century edition, by "A Lover of Philalethes" (1714)

ILLUSTRATIONS: 211-244

NOTES AND REFERENCE SOURCES, 245

NOTE: throughout this book *Kabbalah* refers to the specifically Jewish traditions, while *Qabalah* refers to the broader Hermetic stream that includes Pagan, Christian, Islamic, and Jewish Tree of Life and related geometric spiritual and mystical traditions.

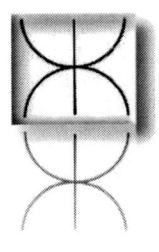

PREFACE

In this second volume of *The Sphere of Art* new methods are offered for sacromagical and theurgic work within the empowered Sphere. These methods are firmly founded in enduring tradition, specifically the Western esoteric or Hermetic tradition that has continued, unbroken, for many centuries. Its roots can be discerned in myths and specific metaphysical works of ancient origin, such as those of the Greek Philosophers, Assyrian, Persian and Egyptian religion, and the all pervasive traditions of the Tree of Life that encompass many expressions, especially the Qabalah that fuses Jewish, Christian, and Islamic mysticism and magic with older and perennial metaphysical traditions. We can think of this immense flow of tradition, seemingly disrupted by militant religion, but in truth well able to resurrect itself through the centuries, as an ancient tree.

There has been considerable vicious pruning by vested interests, but the roots are deep, and the vitality has not diminished, indeed, it has effloresced since the 19th century, in a revival reminiscent of the European Renaissance of the 14th – 17th centuries, both in rediscovery and exposition of occult or magical subjects, and in absurdity and artificiality. In both revivals, that of the occult theosophists and metaphysical philosophers of Renaissance Europe, and that of the ritual occultists, spiritualists, alchemists of the 19th and New Age entrepreneurs of the 20th centuries, there have been some remarkable re-connections to the tree, and steady new growth. These re-connections may be hidden amidst tinsel decoration, but they are discoverable by anyone with common-sense, inspiration, and dedication.

The Efflorescent Tree

The Renaissance philosophers were deeply concerned with Heaven, not necessarily that of the Christian Churches, but the cosmos as an expression of Divine Being. The 19th century occultists were more concerned with individual power, and with shaking off the dross of dogma to bring in evolutionary forces, especially as the true and astounding physical nature of the heavens was finally observed through new telescopes in their era, disposing of an absurd religious strangle-hold that had clung to life for centuries. This impetus continued into the 20th century, and more recently has developed a gradual emphasis upon the roots of the tree. These roots, the spiritual forces of planet Earth as distinct from the heavens, have long been repudiated. Yet the most ancient ancestral sources, and the living indigenous traditions, have all declared the *interior of the planet* to be a source of spiritual transformation. We can continue just a little further with the analogy; the first revival of the Renaissance theosophists revitalized the branches and the sublime crown reaching to the sky and touching the Stars; the second revival of the Victorian occultists explored the vital forces of the trunk; the third phase, which we are still within, untangles and draws nourishment from the roots, so essential to the health of both trunk and branches. Only thus may we reach the Stars.

The *Sphere of Art* offers a simple and comprehensive way of working with roots, trunk, and crown in harmony. This has always been the "secret" way, of course, but the roots were systematically forbidden through a pseudo-tradition of religious propaganda that is now almost defunct.

The practical exercises in this book will work only if you devote your time and energy to learning and practice, and commit to actually doing them. Reading about the concepts is inspiring, but reading itself will not suffice, as it is only a first step. If you follow the methods described, you will have results, moving gradually into deep changes of consciousness. Only after such deep changes within may the outer world be changed; the purifying and transformative forces that you will experience can, and do, make such outer changes. There are no hidden shortcuts, for the practical exercises described here are already shortcuts, and require only repeated dedication of moderate amounts of time in a regular pattern.

There are further levels of this work that have always been taught direct, as they cannot be conveyed in text alone: these further levels are communicated in small groups or classes. This aspect of the tradition is discussed in several places in the following chapters. The methods presented here, however, are complete within themselves, and can be used in your spiritual or sacromagical *Sphere of Art* practice. In this book there is none of the customary obfuscation that is found in older source texts on Qabalah or Alchemy.

How Much Can Be Taught Through Text?

This is a book of possibilities, especially the possibility of transformation and liberation through carefully selected simple and precise methods. My task as author has been to present these methods in ways that can be understood and gradually practiced by the reader or by a group of readers. While fiction is typically a passive entertainment, books on consciousness and on methods of inner transformation require something different; from our initial involvement as readers we can progress to become active participants. Presenting the means for such participation is not easy for an author, as he or she has to find ways by which the reader can develop subtle practices from textual guidance alone. I have been working on this interesting challenge for thirty-five years or more in a series of books, exploring various paths whereby the reader can change consciousness and perception through tried and tested methods. The methods are always tested "in the field" by myself and by groups of experienced students and associates, before they are published.

From the earliest of times, there has been a paradox within text, be it a clay tablet, a papyrus scroll, a printed book, or a display on a flat-screen. Nuances and hyper-levels of meaning often cannot be communicated by text alone. When we consider texts on metaphysics, the Western consciousness can become hopelessly ensnared in increasingly complex and redundant mental speculation. Combine this intellectual obsessiveness with manipulation of vocabulary (rather than communication of meaning), and the reader is propelled further from inner understanding or inspired vision, distanced from the very ideas and truths that are, supposedly, the purpose of the text.

It is well known that ancient mystical, religious, sacromagical sources were often intentionally incomplete. The text was always intended to be a guideline, and to be further elucidated verbally. This method was, originally, due to the difficulty of giving spiritual experiences through text alone: it can occasionally be achieved with poetry, or through those short inspirational statements that are the hallmarks of great spiritual exemplars, but is extremely difficult to convey in prose.

Thus certain material was written down in the sacromagical or theurgic texts of the past, but the methods of *activation* were not. Completion came through individual initiation and enlightenment via direct transmission, beginning with a verbal teaching, but reaching further beyond words.

Over time, the method of incomplete text and verbal teaching became stylized, and people eventually discovered that they could manipulate text to mislead the reader, thus creating an "elite" who had the keys to the real meaning, and an "under-class" who only had the book, or in some cases, such as the early centuries of the Bible, not even that. Such is the basis of the formal book religions; over centuries their esoteric component has rigidified into exoteric dogma and false authority, often enforced by violence. When such rigidity develops, the esoteric component fails to survive, and spiritual vibrancy moves elsewhere, leaving an empty shell of formal politicized religion, or, on a smaller scale, an occult lodge with rules grades and texts, but no inspiration, no living Inner Contacts.

The Scrambled Order

In many alchemical and Qabalistic texts, the *order* of work is intentionally scrambled or misinformed. This later method is derived from systems of symbolism and numeracy, easily presented out of their true order, becoming blinds and baffles for the student. The secret teaching was communicated verbally, and never fully written, always beginning with the correct order for the content used in initial training. Such is true, for example, of the *Aesch Mezareph, Purifying Fire,* text that we explore in several later chapters. It was a book of wonders, containing ways of working with planetary and cosmic forces to catalyze transformation. Published in English from a pseudonymous 18th century translation, presented and annotated by Dr. Wynn Westcott in 1894, and described as "A Chymico-Kabalistic Treatise," it is drawn from the substantial collection Kabala Denudata, assembled by Knorr Von Rosenroth, published in Sulzbach, 1677-1684.

But if you try to do anything as described in the text, if you attempt to take the text literally, it will not work. In his 19th edition, Wynn Westcott advises the reader that there is much intentional confusion and incompletion. The same method of obfuscation was followed in practice by the Hermetic Order of the Golden Dawn that Dr. Westcott helped to found. In subsequent decades, intentionally scrambled esoteric methods and attributes or symbol structures have been idly copied by many who, without experience, unwittingly hand on the confusion to their readers.

It has become standard to say that the more obscure and impossible a magical text, the more powerful and remarkable it must be. This is nonsense: in all practical thaumaturgy, ritual magic, theurgy, or whatever we care to call it, only a clear understanding of our working content will bring results.

The New Way

In the 20th century a small number of writers and teachers on spiritual matters have steadily developed a new way of presentation, in which all the material presented is unambiguous there is no intention of misleading the reader. From such methods, in print and occasionally supported by audio recordings, it is possible to learn and practice so that actual results are achieved. We can do things with our spiritual or sacromagical arts, rather than merely read about them and be puzzled over the content. In the early to mid-20th century, British writers used the phrase "armchair occultists" to describe those who read but do not practice. Today we might say "internet occultists" or "media magicians", who browse endless websites and watch interactive astrological or geometric Platonic diagrams, but do not practice. But there are also many dedicated workers of practical magic and spiritual transformation, more now than at any time in the history of the old Christian and current post-Christian eras.

From the textual, we progress to practice. The practices of meditation, vision, and theurgic or sacromagical rituals, can be undertaken by anyone with some dedication and discipline.

From the practical we pass to inner communion. Consciousness realigns, we attune to new modes of awareness that were not previously possible. It is only at this third stage that the further direct teaching (through shared practice, not mere verbal explanation) is truly effective. We can define the three stages as:

1: Educational, within which textual leads to practical.

2: Experiential, in which practical leads to inner communion and re-alignment.

3: Thaumaturgical and theurgic, in which realignment of consciousness/inner communion leads to on-going dedicated sacromagical work, communicated directly without text.

What is Left Out?

What is left out of this book, therefore, is whatever you will arrive at if you do the practices. The methods come to full fruition within us, and cannot bear such fruit upon the printed page. Beyond the fruition within, there are subtle interactions, teachings, and experiences that can only be shared directly, and cannot be put into text. These deeper experiences can be yours, if you choose to work diligently with the *Purifying Fire*, within the *Sphere of Art*.

R. J. Stewart, Glastonbury, Britain, 2011

INTRODUCTION

This second volume of *The Sphere of Art* offers further techniques and insights into working with *Aesch Mezareph* or *Purifying Fire*. This book is not limited to commentary upon the historical alchemical text of the same name; it is primarily an exploration and expansion of esoteric methods of transformation. Such methods are found not only within the original *Aesch Mezareph*, but in a creative and living sacromagical tradition. As an initiated member of that tradition, I have developed the methods and taught many of them to my students over a number of years. Everything in this book has been worked practically and proven in its own fire of purification. As always, the material offered here is intended for contemporary use, for the 21st century and onwards. It does not hark back to a romanticized pseudo-ancient world of Alchemy or Qabalah, druids and magicians, and does not hide behind obscure terminology or linguistics.

It is sometimes forgotten that the source texts available to us in the spiritual or magical traditions were intended to be contemporary...they were created or assembled for the present, for their own time, and further intended as gifts of wisdom to the uncertain future rather than as sources of escape into the abandoned past. The requirements of each era change, and what had to be hidden due to persecution in the past, may now be carefully revealed. Amused disbelief today is preferable to torture or prosecution. In addition, I do not subscribe to the unhealthy idea that only an elite group of people may practice spiritual transformation, so that other kind of "secrecy", founded in a false occult superiority tottering upon individual fear and insecurity, can play no part in a book of this sort.

The Three Sources of Aesch Mezareph in this Book

There are three sources for the term *Aesch Mezareph* in this book. The Anglicized spelling of the original Hebrew or Aramaic phrase should probably be *Ash Metzareph*, though this is seldom seen. The first source, widely available in reprint and on the internet, is a complex Kabbalistic and alchemical text of uncertain date, but unquestionably with origins prior to its 17th century Latin edition, drawing upon a Hebrew or Aramaic source that is now presumably lost. The title of the 19th century English publication of this text, by Dr. Wynn Westcott, has established the current spelling. As Westcott himself said about this historical book, anyone trying to work with its methods as they are written will fail to achieve anything.

It is likely, given the methods and secrecy of the early Kabbalistic groups and alchemists, that the original was a set of teachings or aphorisms first communicated verbally, later transcribed, and having marginal annotations added that were gradually incorporated into an increasingly confused, and confusing, text. The process of unwittingly incorporating annotations from a hand-written manuscript into what would eventually become the "definitive" text, when printed at a much later date, sometimes centuries after the original was penned, is well-known in Kabbalistic sources [1]. As discussed shortly, there are other reasons why the historical text *Aesch Mezareph* may be unclear or, as it stands, unworkable without special interpretation and elucidation. Such unworkable natures are rife in alchemical and Kabbalistic/Qabalistic texts, so in this book, for the contemporary reader and practitioner, I have aimed for clarity and simplicity.

The second source is, of course, the phrase itself, which means *Fire of Purification*. *Ash/Aesch* is fire, and *Metzareph/Mezareph* is purification, as in metallic purification within a heated crucible or forge. Thus it is term of metallurgy, Alchemy, and spiritual purification, from both a time and a consciousness wherein the three were not separate. Both words, in this context, have Hebrew or Aramaic origins, and their roots permeate a number of languages. This *Purifying Fire* is required in all processes of transformation, from the physical to the spiritual, but the present context refers specifically to the use of subtle fire within the *Sphere of Art*, a sacromagical technique described in detail in

Volume One. The practical use of attuned Purifying Fire, *Aesch Mezareph*, is the main subject of this second volume.

Some significant clues are found in the historic text, but the methods that I offer here for working with the Purifying Fire (themselves refined in that same fire) are new, and have been carefully developed for contemporary use. This book is not a detailed study of the historic text, therefore, but an exploration and elucidation of a method hidden within that text, a text that contains several alchemical transformative techniques, sometimes randomized and enfolded within one-another.

The method offered herein comes not solely from the historic text, but from a living initiatory tradition. The source text is an intentionally scrambled set of notes and hyper-references such as was typical of many early Qabalistic and alchemical treatises. That older way of working is not used here, though a basic expansion of some of the hyper-references in *Aesch Mezareph* is offered in Chapter Seven, where the first chapter of the source text is partially elucidated.

This provides insights into how such material was devised and was intended to be read by early teachers of the tradition. My short elucidation is not intended to be authoritative or complete, but is offered to demonstrate certain concepts and to give subtle clues for further inspiration. In this I cannot better the words of the unknown author of *Aesch Mezareph*, centuries past, who writes: *"Thus I have delivered to thee the key to unlock many secret gates, and have opened the door to the inmost adyta of Nature. But if anyone hath placed those things in another order, I shall not contend with him, inasmuch as all systems tend to the one truth"*.

The third source is a gravestone in a quiet Somerset graveyard, bearing the faded inscription "Aesch Mezereph", a slightly variant spelling, possibly a slip on the part of an executor or stone-mason. Why did Alfred Ronald Heaver, the hidden Glastonbury Adept (1900-1980) have this obscure line, along with a verse from the book of Isaiah, on his grave? As a Qabalist and mystic, it would certainly be appropriate, as all inner transformation is a process of purification. During a discussion in the late 1960's, and in subsequent letters, ARH stated "Everyone thinks they need more power, when what is really needed is more purification". Variants on this would arise in his conversations and correspondence during the latter years of his life. Not Power, but Purification. This might be misinterpreted, of course, as some prim Christianizing of the life forces, but that would be far indeed from its true meaning!

As a young man, ARH used subtle forces to effect a seemingly miraculous self-healing in the 1920's when he was told that he only had a short time to live, after injuries to his spine incurred during the First World War [2]. My understanding is that he used *Aesch Mezareph*, the Purifying Fire. From his cryptic conversations and inferences in the 1970's, I gradually developed new methods, over a long period of time, eventually appearing as *The Sphere of Art.* These methods, if carefully followed, will focus the Purifying Fire naturally in a direct and harmonious way.

The inscription on ARH's gravestone is a typical cryptic clue. We might summarize his message as "purify yourself with fire as did I and while you are so involved, there are hints in a historic text to which you should pay attention". This approach is typical of ARH, who laid everything out in the open in a concise concentrated manner that had to be grasped by the recipient quickly, for there were few second chances. We must always remember, therefore, that the act of purification itself is of far greater significance than merely studying a text about Alchemy or Qabalah. The texts often provide clues, but the purification is something that we must do for ourselves.

All three sources, the historic text, the Hebrew phrase, and the inscription, come down to one concentrated theme...work diligently with the Purifying Fire. This book, the second volume of *The Sphere of Art*, describes in detail certain specific sacromagical and simple alchemical practices that can be done *within* the Sphere of Art. They are partly developed from subtle clues in the *Aesch Mezareph* source text, and partly from the deep ongoing impetus of the living initiatory stream itself. The result is a set of methods that are an elucidation of inner teachings, enabling results from working with the fire of purification. Paradoxically, when we have let go of the idea of gaining more power, and have passed through the fire of purification, we will have whatever power we need, rather than any spurious illusory power that we may have originally desired.

While the source material that I have drawn upon can be described as "alchemical" in a broad sense, the practices may also be described as "theurgic". The terms theurgy and thaumaturgy, originally deriving from the ancient Greek, were used by certain mystics and occultists, including ARH, in an attempt to side-step the unsavory aspects of the widespread popularization and trivializing of Magic.

In the first Chapter, we will explore the nature and practice of Theurgy, Thaumaturgy, and dedicated Sacromagical work, with special reference to *The Sphere of Art.*

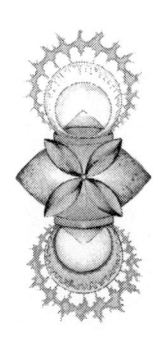

CHAPTER ONE

THEURGY AND THAUMATURGY, HIGH AND LOW MAGIC

Theurgy and Thaumaturgy

The perennial esoteric practical traditions are sometimes described as *theurgic*. In the term "practical" we include all methods that lead toward change, providing they are undertaken consciously, with the intention of seeking change. Theurgy is by no means limited to formal rituals with robes and altars: these adjuncts are merely the costumes and settings for the true theurgy, and can take many forms, visible and invisible.

In this book the terms *theurgy* and *sacromagical* refer to techniques and traditions of spiritual magic. Such arts are practiced to bring the consciousness into a new state, to transform the entire being, and eventually to transform the entire world, albeit one step at a time. So if you are interested in spells for egocentric power, cursing, communing with deceased spirits and so forth, this book is not for you, and you will find it boring. The methods herein require discipline, commitment, and compassion...without compassion all spiritual magic ultimately will fail, no matter what short term results may be attained. The interplay between theurgy and thaumaturgy has been explored in many books, but has often been somewhat misrepresented. Such misrepresentation in 19th and early 20th century presentations is usually due to an overlay from dogmatic religion such as Christianity, as if this were the only possible avenue for theurgy. There is, however, a significant body of early Christian theurgic material, often deriving from Neo-Platonic sources. We are fortunate to have some theurgic texts from such ancient sources, offering us insights into the theurgic philosophy and metaphysics of the ancestral cultures [37].

High and Low Magic

For many years there has been a repeated distinction made, in various texts and practices from many sources, between "low" and "high" magic. Low magic is supposedly a dangerous morass of suspect practices, while high magic is supposedly reputable and noble, though often incomprehensible; its glamorous incomprehensibility is often most attractive to those who would rather browse than practice.

We find this dualism of low and high magic repeated in a somewhat modified way in modern use of the terms *theurgy* and *thaumaturgy*, as if thaumaturgy, working in nature through magic, is in some way a lower "opposite" of the higher theurgy, working in spiritual dimensions through magic. Theurgy and thaumaturgy are definitions of *movement*: the first moves consciousness and energy into spiritual dimensions through sacromagical practices, especially ritual, while the second moves consciousness and energy in the polar direction, into nature, though sacromagical practices. In theurgic practices, a response is sought from higher orders of consciousness...originally from the gods and goddesses, or from emanations of the Divine Being. In thaumaturgic practices a reaction is sought, from lesser orders of consciousness, resonating into the world of nature. If you are deeply involved in such practices, rather than a superficial dabbler, you cannot truly practice one without the other. Certain thaumaturgical effects, however, can be achieved without a theurgic approach, and we will return to these shortly.

If we take time to examine magical arts in their various forms handed down in tradition, folklore, definitive texts as distinct from superficial derivatives, and through the various initiatory streams, we soon find that the dualistic definitions of so-called high and low magic are untenable. Folkloric magic (low) often holds echoes of the profound spiritual traditions of our ancestors, while sophisticated texts from occult orders (high) are sometimes replete with appalling ignorance and absurd nonsense. Added to this are the innumerable vexed problems of ancient texts, frequently revealing a mixture of both "high" and "low" magical practices, whisked together uncritically and seemingly at random. This uncritical mix is not entirely due to the presumed ignorance of the ancients, but has a more complex foundation.

The thaumaturgical marvels of the ancients, such as those attributed to various saints, masters, and metaphysical philosophers, were said to occur due to higher spiritual forces directing the natural world through the ethical practices and qualities of the individual concerned, ultimately as a process of *mediation*. Similar effects were supposed to be possible through an unethical use of coercion and through pacts with unhealthy parasitic familiar spirits: this is where the idea of thaumaturgy divorced from theurgy, mentioned above, has gained new impetus in popular books on magic.

If we research and contemplate, we will find that the real distinction between high and low magic is one of ethics, or the lack thereof, and not one of methodology or streams of tradition. All magical arts can be employed in all possible ways, for they are tools, not ends in themselves. In this book we are concerned with practices that are ethical and have a compassionate foundation. Co-operation is always more productive and longer-lived than coercion.

Inside the Activated Sphere of Art

Inside the activated Sphere of Art subtle forces that are often called "low" are transformed toward "high". A process of *fusion* of subtle forces is employed. Energies that might not normally meet come together to merge as new consciousness, new expressions within nature. As we, ourselves, are the content of the Sphere, such new expressions occur first within ourselves, and from our simple starting place, resonate outwards into the world.

In modern science this potential for transformation or conversion of energy has been utilized in many ways in our development of electricity, so models of energy conversion are relatively well known, and have many practical applications that we use daily without being aware of their origins, or, in some examples, even of their existence.

In the Sphere of Art conversion of energy is empowered in two ways, by the rising UnderWorld telluric forces of our sacred planet, which are simultaneously Earthly and Stellar, and by the descending Stellar forces from the greater cosmos. The fusion of these two within the Sphere creates a third spiritual power...the New Sun.

As we might expect in an era when the sacred Earth is abused and its spiritual potential repudiated, it is the telluric UnderWorld and Earth Light energies that are of deep relevance to us at this time. If we are able to work with the Rising Light forces effectively, much of the stellar response is guaranteed. During this process, psychic energies employed in the so-called "low" magical arts of thaumaturgy are no longer fragmentary or dissociated, but are brought into specific roles and functions. In this manner they come to serve our "high" magic or theurgy, coming into harmony and balance. Understanding something of the dynamics of this process is essential for work with Aesch Mezareph, Purifying Fire.

In old fashioned terminology such dynamics would be firmly described as a process of spiritual redemption, and in the most profound ancestral traditions such redemption can only begin within the UnderWorld. Today we might say that it occurs due to interaction with the Earth Light, that transformative spiritual power inherent within our planet... we should always remember that the nearest Star is just beneath our feet. At this level of sacromagical work we set aside all propagandist nonsense regarding the Earth as evil or the UnderWorld as "hell": the time is long overdue to dispose of such ignorance or intentional manipulative conditioning.

The Sacromagical Process of Redemption and Evolution

There is a process whereby the dissociated and often random psychic and sexual forces that can support unhealthy or parasitic entities in crude unethical magic are both redeemed and evolved. This process is external in the sense that redemptive forces work as catalysts on all that they touch, and internal in the sense they work on our own imbalances within. Typically for us, as humans, the adjustment (often associated with the spiritual power embodied in the traditional trump or emblem of Justice) occurs after death and before rebirth, but it can also be consciously achieved in one lifetime through discipline and dedicated spiritual work. This is often described as an intentional acceleration of the evolutionary impetus, or "Shortened Way".

The words Redemption and Evolution have much unfortunate baggage attached to them, so some basic definitions, for the purposes of this book, will be helpful to us.

Redemption, regardless of special religious definitions, means to re-deem, repay, or give back something that was originally received. Thus you can redeem a loan of something by giving it back, or your own loan or gift or loss can be redeemed by something returned to you. Through religious influence redemption has become associated with both pernicious dogma and insightful teachings, regarding the inner human condition of balance and how it might be improved.

Evolution means to roll-out (Latin: *evolvare*). In sacromagical arts it has a further definition of spiritual movement from the Earth toward the Stars, often termed the Evolutionary Stream. This Evolutionary Stream is balanced by an Involutionary Stream, from the Stars toward the Earth. While the twin streams are a deeply rooted aspect of the older spiritual traditions, they are redefined by contemporary physics as those radiant measurable forces emitted by the Earth, and those received from the cosmos, a vast spectrum of energies that is still being catalogued. The two sets of forces, those emitted from the planet and those coming into it and sometimes penetrating deep within, are in constant array...we live within them and would have no life without them.

In Bardic or Druidic tradition the evolutionary and involutionary forces were perceived spiritually, described poetically, and were said to be embodied by the Red and White Dragons. [3]. We could also add that observation of nature has always shown that there is an upward or outward movement in the growth of plants or the expansion of species in Spring and Summer, cycling toward a downward or reducing movement, in

Autumn and Winter, returning to rebirth with the new year. Such cycles are at the heart of many myths and legends, and deeply rooted within most religions, ranging from observation of nature to contemplation of the galaxy and cosmos.

There is no value judgment in the concepts of the Evolutionary and Involutionary Streams. Evolution and Involution are equally sacred forces, one moving from the center of the Earth through Moon, Sun and Planets, out toward the Stars, the other coming in from the cosmos. Involution should not be confused with devolution or retrogression. When this twofold polarized movement is identified as the source of birth, death, and rebirth, we can come to understand that there is no evolution without involution...to *evolve* we must become *involved*.

Alchemy and Evolution

In alchemical tradition there is a foundational concept of the *evolution* of the metals, typically, but by no means exclusively, from lead toward gold. Other evolutionary or accelerated energies are said to manifest as described in the well-known stories of the Philosopher's Stone, and the Red and White Projections, described as powders that catalyze transformation. In our exploration of the *Aesch Mezareph* within the Sphere of Art, we are not concerned with the upward conversion of metals for material benefit, nor are we subsumed into a merely psychological model of Alchemy. Both interpretations are, in essence, materialist, and can be (depending upon interpretation and presentation) in many ways inadequate. As there is a huge body of literature on each, there seems little purpose in adding further content here.

In the esoteric alchemical traditions, of which there are several sharing a perennial common core, the evolution of the metals is likened to the redemptive process in humanity, through which we are transformed away from confusion ignorance and isolation toward balance knowledge and harmony with all beings. Many of the attributes of this process are established through the traditional forces ascribed to the Wanderers or Seven Planets, and at a deeper esoteric level to all ten Emanations of the Tree of Life.

As an example, Saturn, associated with lead, can contain and limit certain potentially damaging chaotic energies within; the energies themselves are not "evil" but if they are imbalanced or misplaced can certainly cause difficulties for the individual and for those in association with him or her. Saturn often seems, to the uninitiated, like an inhibiting or testing and challenging energy in the natal chart, yet it is ultimately protective and transformative, just as lead, the metal of Saturn, is used today to shield against radiation. Saturn, at its deepest level, is the Vessel or Mother Power of the Tree of Life, Universal Understanding, the Third Emanation, containing all, drawing all into herself for potential renewal. See Figure One (The Tree of Life)

We find this process of Evolution described in our historical text, *Aesch Mezareph* in three modes: the first is in the context of the Emanations of the Tree of Life, the second is shown as the Evolution of the Metals, and the third as transformative forces working through the natural orders of life...animals, birds, fishes, and so forth, albeit in the form of hybrid living creatures, typical to alchemical mystical and prophetic texts. That the spiritual forces may appear in this specific triple order is no coincidence. The Emanations of the Tree of Life come first as they are the cosmic templates or Platonic archetypes of creation. Next these forces, which for us on Earth are typified by the traditional septenary of Sun, Moon, and Planets, are mirrored directly within the body of the planet, from the Stars through the Solar System into the Earth, where they manifest substantially as the metals. To expand from the Seven to the Ten of the Tree of Life, we add further primal planetary substances, which will be described in our later chapters.

Only after this mirroring in the Earth, the UnderWorld, do we find the forms of Nature in the original *Aesch Mezareph*, as in other alchemical source texts, in a typical shape-changing sequence such as is found in folk tales, magical ballads, and primal sacromagical practices world-wide.

All three of these may be understood not as mere allegories of the human transformation process, but as direct energies, as forces of catalysis, *within and of themselves*. This direct energetic interaction between human and other orders of life is missing from a merely psychological interpretation of alchemical texts; such texts were never merely symbolic of human mental and emotional processes, though there is little doubt that they can be applied, in a somewhat limited manner, to represent such processes.

The foundation of all spiritual arts of transformation, including Alchemy and Qabalistic mysticism as combined in our source text, is that potent transformative processes are *already present* within all things, from the simplest single celled organism to the burning radiant Stars of the cosmos. As the perennial wisdom traditions teach us, such processes may be found consciously in humanity.

The transformative processes are never the solely-owned property of the human brain, or limited to adaptive or conditioned patterns within the psyche, but permeate all existence. They are more accurately understood as a continuum of *movement* from one condition to another, and when we experience this and contemplate it, we discover that many of the standard value-judgments, such as higher/lower, are relativistic and thus cannot be applied as absolutes.

This poses an interesting moral dilemma that can be confusing or even disempowering for some people, as absolutes are often easier to understand, and relative interactions without moral absolutes can be used as excuses for inertia or indifference. Providing we hold to the idea of a compassionate involvement that leads to mutual co-operative evolution, we can steadily grow beyond such dilemmas.

The sacromagical reasoning of *Aesch Mezareph*, in keeping with classic alchemical philosophy, is that *all things evolve, and all things can be redeemed from a state of confusion and pain toward a state of balance and harmony. The redemption process intervenes in the evolutionary process and accelerates it;* but only under special circumstances, and only in response to conscious recognition. Such intervention is familiar in a dogmatic religious context as the much propagandized and deeply harmful manipulative dualistic ideas of sin and salvation. It is also found in a more positive form in the mystical context of spiritual transformation through grace.

Beyond Dualism: The Threefold Interaction

The Sphere of Art and related practices of the Purifying Fire bring a third concept and set of players into the seemingly dualistic interaction described above. In keeping with alchemical tradition and UnderWorld esoteric traditions, the third set is that of *any evolving order of life* (other than human), from mineral to biological, to spiritual or metaphysical, from planetary to stellar. Typical alchemical methods involve the metals, apparently evolving from lead through a classic planetary sequence toward gold, or even transforming in one seemingly miraculous leap. Alchemy may also involve working with plant materials, or combinations of plant and metal transformation and experiment. In the methods described in this book, we focus primarily but not exclusively upon the metals or minerals and their planetary and spiritual resonances and counterparts.

In the initiatory traditions we are given to understand that if we can interact with the spiritual forces of such mysterious evolution, they will intervene and accelerate our own evolution. To this end we are invited to remember that we have within us these same metals and substances, in our blood and bones, and that we are composed of their subtle energetic forces, as embodied by the Planets and the Emanations of the Tree of Life that inform and empower the Solar System, and hence the Planets and the Metals in the Earth.

The Threefold Interaction can be defined simply as follows:

1: Humanity seeks consciously to transform itself, and so begins to build a relationship with spiritual forces of evolution.

2: Spiritual forces of evolution, as shown upon the Tree of Life, are combined with a further relationship to *any other evolving set or order of life*.

3: Any other evolving set or order of life includes, but is not limited to, the metals, the living creatures, the faery and spirit races, the plant world, the angelic realms, the Inner Temples, and so on. The process is one of interaction and catalysis.

The results, and the subtle qualities and properties, of such threefold alliance, will vary according to the partners in the relationship. Hence the text of *Aesch Mezareph* advises us that we can relate through the Emanations mirrored within ourselves as the human participants, and further interact with a third component, in one of the other worlds, especially the mineral, or that of myriad orders of life in Nature. Other Qabalistic and alchemical texts offer similar advice, on potential union with various orders of spiritual beings and angels, while the folkloric faery tradition employs a threefold alliance of Human, Faery, and Living Creature [4]. (See Figure Seventeen)

Curiously, the historic text titled *Aesch Mezareph* does not speak of angels or Archangels, or other orders of spiritual beings, though it does describe magical creatures as forms of transformation that may be observed, metaphorically, during Alchemy. It may be that the original text belongs to a school that did not work with spiritual intermediaries, preferring to focus directly upon the Emanations and their relationship to the spiritual forces of the metals. It seems more likely, given the widespread use of angelic and spiritual communion in the esoteric tradition, that these aspects of the Tree of Life were intentionally omitted, especially as the interactions possible through Archangelic or angelic communion, were originally closely guarded secrets. A clue to this pattern might be found in the various injunctions found in many texts against working with angelic names, and we will return to this somewhat paradoxical theme later…why list them, describe them, and then say we must not work with them?

While our everyday outer life relies mainly on gaining experience through human interaction alone, the potential Threefold Interaction, described above, opens us to new levels of awareness that are typically excluded from human experience. In our modernist post-Christian culture we have become painfully aware of humanity's rejection of the natural world in favor of machines and media simulacra, yet this hostility to nature, for which we are only now discovering the price, is but a small part of our real rejection and lack of interaction.

The principle and practice of threefold interaction, as described, carries with it some significant ideas about redemption and liberation, for it is not human-centric. The liberation and evolution is through *mutual interaction* whereby all parties, all sets, all orders of being, benefit one another.

This interaction is undertaken within the activated Sphere of Art. The energetic field of the Sphere is analogous to the sealed physical vessel described in so many alchemical texts, within which the metals are evolved or transformed and other redemptive processes occur. The basic methods of creating and activating the Sphere of Art are described in detail in Volume One, book and audio CD, The Sphere of Art.

While general evolutionary movement is found in the broadcast seeds of interaction in nature and in daily life, the containment of the Sphere and its precise focusing of subtle forces substantially enhance and accelerate transformation.

In this second volume we will explore some of the spiritual principles that can be applied in Sphere of Art work. If we are able to transform our thought-processes away from inherent dualism toward a fluid relativity, we begin truly to change not only ourselves, but the world in which we live. This is the mystery of redemption as a living force, rather than as religious dogma.

What is Given Back? The Redemption of Energy

In a crude or dogmatic religious interpretation, redemption is often about paying your dues for bad behavior in order that you may escape punishment or damnation. Typically a special spiritual power is invoked, whereby the human is saved through intervention, as in the various religious traditions worldwide. At its best this is a beautiful teaching about higher orders of compassion aiding misguided humanity, at its worst it can be a tool of manipulation through fear. But what exactly is *redeemed*? There can only be one effective answer to this: *energy*. The soul, so often referred to, so seldom adequately defined, is a field of energy. Different traditions describe it in various ways.

In the perennial esoteric traditions, the soul is regarded as a field of energy that evolves through experience: it may come into more than one birth by building a series of physical bodies through a long cycle of reincarnations, or it may move in the polar direction beyond physical expression, and no longer reincarnate. The soul is a resonance or harmonic that builds between the originative Spirit or Being, and a manifest form or Body. It is another Third, such as those found in the threefold interactions described above, resonating between the First and Last, the Who and the What, the Spirit and the Form. Souls have to grow and evolve…they are not finite creations owned by an angry or possessive deity, no matter how often we are told this told by the Book Religions.

In the Fire Temple tradition associated with our Sphere of Art practices, we work within the Sphere to receive into ourselves certain spiritual evolutionary forces (energy) in a clear and harmonious pattern. In a simple sense we could say that it is not we who are being "saved" by an external entity, as in the religious model, but that when we discover how to go half-way, to a threshold of consciousness and energy, *we are given back our true and original condition of Being*. We become what we always have been, through redemption, through our willing reception of that which is *given back to us*. Of course for this to work, even in a minor way, we have to understand what we gave away, lost, or lent in the first place. This understanding comes to us not solely from an inner sense of longing or loss, but from a truly compassionate sense of the suffering of others.

What Did we Lose, and Who Gives it Back?

The Map and the Territory

Our various spiritual philosophical and metaphysical traditions advise that we do not understand, or participate in, our original and true relationship to the cosmos in which we live. While many traditions promote antagonistic dualism in this respect, we could use instead the classic allegory of being *lost*. Our condition is like that of someone who wakes up one morning with no memory, in a strange territory into which they have mysteriously wandered during their sleep in the night.

With no memory or knowledge of this territory our person is lost and he or she begins to wander further, accumulating what they hope is accurate knowledge of their surroundings. Gradually this interaction, with iincreasingly polarized thoughts and feelings, accumulates a weight, a presence, a mass, of its own. Eventually it becomes the world for our individual, who incrementally substitutes a map for the territory. The map is "known", while the territory itself becomes increasingly "strange" as the individual increasingly lives through the map of what he/she "knows". By doing so he/she becomes progressively lost while enfolded within the illusion of increasing knowledge.

This simple allegory, of which there are many variants in spiritual or philosophical traditions, gives us a better sense of our condition than calling it fallen sinful doomed and so forth. In this *lost* condition, the individual can make choices not just about how he or she *interprets* the territory, but about how to *interact* with it. Such choices can be ethical or unethical, and this dialectic of choice especially comes into play in our interactions with others who are equally lost and also trying to map the territory to acquire their own set of "meanings".

Most issues come down to questions such as: do we help others who are lost, do we take advantage of them, or do we repudiate them and continue to develop our own map? Extreme examples are found when individuals or self-serving collectives seek to impose their map upon others. Such collective impositions can gather enormous energy permeating and dominating the psyche of nations; the 20th century amply demonstrated this with surges of Fascism and Communism. Earlier eras, which still have a strong presence today, generated the collective impositions, maps, and imprints of dogmatic religion, that continue to dominate in many parts of the world, but are currently fighting one another to the death. We are witnessing the death throes of the Book religions, though this will be a long drawn out process.

What we have described above, waking up in an unknown territory and the concomitant need to build a map, is, of course, that which happens when we are born and live through our life cycle with little or no conscious spiritual awareness. When we die we leave the territory of the manifest life, but most of us will try to hold onto the artificial map. Eventually the map is dissolved and forgotten, and we come at last into rebirth, with our memory cleansed. Thus we come again to the territory, albeit with our understanding of it limited or occluded, and we begin the process anew.

The Tree of Life Replaces the Map

Through spiritual practices, however, it is gradually possible to view and comprehend the territory directly, rather than struggle to create and maintain a superimposed map that stands between. Many spiritual disciplines consist, at first, of deconstructing the existing conditioned map; it can be undone rapidly through catharsis, or steadily and intentionally replaced by a glyph or relational map such as the Tree of Life. The Tree replaces the randomly assembled or consensually conditioned map with a hyper-map of qualities and subtle energies that stand behind the outer interactions and circumstances. Thus it moves consciousness in stages toward the territory itself.

These stages are inherent within us, yet need to be consciously activated, and are shown by the Paths and the Emanations of the Tree of Life. Figure One shows the Tree of Life with the harmonious Axis Mundi Path system that was developed in Italy from Platonic and Qabalistic sources, and eventually represented as early hand-painted tarot images, predating any printed decks of cards. The Axis Mundi or Middle Pillar is the natural, relativistic, sequence of Earth, Moon, Sun, and Stars, that Renaissance theosophy and metaphysics drew, at some risk, from the ancient pagan perennial spiritual traditions.

By comparison the so-called "standard" or "authoritative" path attributes to tarot trumps are an intentionally scrambled order used as a blind by 19th century occultists, yet they are repeatedly published by copyists without thought or question. Tarot plays no part in traditional Jewish Kabbalah, though there is some implication that many of the traditional tarot *images* have parallels in Biblical scenes. Similar proto-tarot images are found in the medieval Merlin texts of Geoffrey of Monmouth, that substantially predate the earliest known painted or printed images [5]. Such images have been used allegorically for centuries in traditional wisdom stories, and contain further spiritual and ethical implications for meditation.

What we are given back during the process of redemption is the ability to relate directly to the territory as it really is. This is the greatest gift that we mysteriously lost, that is returned to us through spiritual transformation by agencies of love and compassion. Yet the loving compassionate powers will not, and cannot, give forth until we have purified ourselves by the inner disciplines and transformations; the *Aesch Mezareph* text describes the process clearly for those who are able to read it.

There is no value judgment in this process, for we cannot come to Mercy on the Tree until we have been purified by Severity. We could also say, along with Shakespeare, that the quality of Mercy will inevitably release into a ground that is rightly prepared for it, and will always come after Severity, and not be ultimately held back. Portia's famous speech on the nature of Mercy and Severity in The Merchant of Venice has excellent Qabalistic reasoning: *"The Quality of Mercy is not strained..?"* wherein "strained" is Elizabethan poetic English for constrained, or restricted.

It is not without good reason that spiritual enlightenment is often described as returning home, rediscovering the already known, and remembering. The map is dissolved and we come at last into the territory that we have always occupied but could never fully perceive, because of the map or maps that intervened.

Our cycle of lives involves forgetting, coming into birth, being lost. Thus we perceive the territory only according to our repeated attempts to map it. Sometimes such maps are carried over, at least in part, from life to life, hence those tendencies in the natal chart that must be sublimated through experience in each lifetime. This carrying over of the map can give many insights into the much misrepresented idea of *karma* as individual fate. Thus the Wheels of Fortune or of Justice do not just spin us around or punish us for our folly, but repeatedly pass us through certain occluded parts of the map, bringing the occlusion to our awareness, until we are free of all attachment to them. It is not the act of violence alone that brings a "karmic" effect...it is the consciousness behind that act.

The Enfolding and Interleaved Territories

Our allegory can be extended further: when we first awaken and discover that we are lost, not knowing how or why, our territory is limited to that which is immediate and close. We are often fearful of any movement beyond a small circle around us. We seek to relate to what is directly in front of us, and to build a body of knowledge about that, excluding all else. This is our relationship to, and our incrementally increasing map of, the manifest or material world. Many people go no further than this immediate territory, yet it interacts with other territories that enfold it in all directions; we all know this at a deep non-verbal level of awareness. We cannot feel lost without some inner sense of another perception, another awareness, in which we know that we can ultimately find the real territory, and that it will no longer be strange and frightening. To know that we are lost, we must have some sense of a previous condition in which our understanding was different. This manifests as our deepest intuitions that life is not what we are told, not what we might think, and not as imposed upon us by collective or consensual maps.

Some seek to reduce the territory to as small and controllable a zone as possible, rejecting the natural world in favor of a simulated "controlled" environment. Yet even those who severely limit themselves are occasionally aware of enfolding and interleaving further territories, though they seek to explain them only in terms of the immediate. This syndrome is at its most obvious in the determination that everything must and will have either a material or a psychological explanation. Curiously, it is often those who are sensitive to the further territories that fight the hardest to limit all human knowledge to the manifest, the immediate, and the defensive simulacra that abound within modernism.

As individuals we have varying awareness of the enfolding and interleaved territories, which are the realms of consciousness and energy that create and supply the manifest world...our "known and mapped" territory.

Figure Two (The Three Worlds of Moon Sun Star) is a simple model of how such enfolding manifests in a planetary sense. It is not intended as a literal map, but as a conceptual tool: the world of the Stars or cosmos enfolds all, the world of the Sun enfolds the Planets, and the world of the Moon enfolds the Earth that is within all three enfoldments. Thus while three concentric spheres do not correspond to the physical cosmos as studied in astronomy, they accurately describe the condition and location of our planet Earth and Moon, within the Solar System, within the cosmos. The conceptual model of Earth and Moon within Solar System, Solar System within Stellar Universe can thus be shown by three interlinked or concentric spheres, without conflicting with astronomical data. This enfolded or nested territory map is extremely helpful in meditation, offering us a relative sense of Place that brings liberation from dualism and isolation.

Explanations of Spiritual Awareness and Transformation

The esoteric traditions teach that there are further interleaved or nested territories in metaphysical relationship with one another. This is somewhat similar to certain concepts of quantum mechanics that have arisen in the 20th century, though it must be remembered that modern physics has merely added abstruse mathematics to concepts and models that have existed for millenniums in the esoteric and philosophical traditions. We will not evolve in our spiritual or sacromagical work if we rest upon the naïve idea that it can all be explained by modern physics, just as in the early 20th century it was incorrectly, albeit enthusiastically, assumed that it could all explained by psychology.

In truth, spiritual awareness and transformation cannot be explained at all, for they must first be experienced. Better, then, to explain ways toward that experience, so we may all have it for ourselves.

A much practiced analogy is that of the difference between a description and explanation of any object, say a tree, and actually encountering that object. This is a well-known philosophical discussion that has been explored in many ways through the centuries.

If we have not encountered a tree, no amount of explanation will substitute. If we have encountered a tree, explanation after the event will not enhance or intensify the essence of the encounter...and may eventually put a simulated model between ourselves and our original experience.

This same problem is expressed by Wagner, the amanuensis of Faustus, in Goethe's drama, who complains that art is so long and life is short. This complaint is satirical, but highly effective as a meditation. Goethe based his satire upon a famous aphorism of the classical Greek doctor Hippocrates that is often quoted in alchemical contexts:

> *Life is short,*
> *The art long,*
> *Opportunity fleeting,*
> *Experiment fallible,*
> *Judgment difficult.*

This aphorism is more than a witty comment, for it relates to the Emanations of the Tree of Life.

The ancients used a model in which the seven traditional Planets described the enfolding territories, and had further resonances or affinities within human consciousness; thus Mercury was of thought, Venus of emotions, and so forth. A version of this model is shown in our Figure Three (Seven Planets Enfolding). The orbits of the physical Planets are indeed the cosmic territories or neighborhoods within which our manifest

Earth lives...for all are orbiting in a dynamic relationship around the Sun. Such models do not demand belief in a geocentric system, and they do not imply that the Earth is the center of anything other than our *sense of place*. Thus planet Earth is our *locus* or central point, our relative starting point for identity, as it orbits around the Sun, and as the Sun moves within the Galaxy.

Dissolving Map, Redeeming Mind

When we begin to relate to the territory as it really is, we swiftly begin to lose our limited map. This can be a fearful experience or a joyous one, depending on our individual training, preparation and understanding. To be cast loose without the map that you need for stability is to be at risk of going mad in unknown territory, while to throw the map away willingly in full awareness is to embrace risk and enter a new condition of sanity.

Redemption, when given to us, is the power to relate directly to the territory, and to perceive that it is an enfolded or nested set of many territories one within the other; enfolding all is Unity or Being, out of which the nested territories have manifested.

Rather than reject the manifest world we can choose to participate in its transformation into wholeness. The individual mind that has struggled to map the territory is vibrantly subsumed into the Unity of Mind embracing all territories. When all individual forms of consciousness come to relate directly to the territory, the totality is transformed, and is uplifted, evolved, into a new condition. Paradoxically, it was there all along, but we were not able to perceive it. Hence our many difficult religious and philosophical themes relating to being "fallen" exiled or cast out of Heaven, and the clumsy, or subtle and often deceitful, explanations that so easily become dogma, yet can never replace spiritual experience.

The Childhood Explorer

This lost territory model also describes childhood. When we are newly born, and during our young years usually up to about the age of seven, we may frequently perceive the territory as it truly is. The infant seeks to learn about the manifest world but also lives in the un-manifest territories that enfold it. As is well known, an infant begins to develop a map very early; much of our younger life consists of friction between the map that we are developing and the maps offered to us, sometimes imposed upon us, by adults. In the individual who continues to think, to wonder, to question, such friction between internal and external maps, or individual and consensual models of supposed reality, seldom ceases.

Religions and spiritual traditions offer their various maps of the enfolded or interleaved territories; some appear to be liberating maps that encourage individual enlightenment, while others appear to be impositions to keep us under control. In the initiatory traditions such maps are understood as being useful only as interim descriptions, helping us to move away from a confused and lost state, beyond the limited repetitious maps of narrow territory, into a greater perspective. In the deeper Mysteries the initiatory maps themselves are progressively disposed of step by step, as the initiate comes into a more direct perception of the enfolding interleaved territories.

Pins on the Map: The Inner Temples

A significant role is played by those special constructs that are found in certain mystery schools or initiatory traditions. Sometimes loosely defined as "thought-forms", such constructs are what we term the Inner Temples and the timeless Inner Convocation[6]. More than mere thought-forms, they are locations of energy and consciousness that are held together by many conscious beings, creating and sustaining shared transcendent images, unlimited by the cycles of time and nature.

A metaphysical definition of the Inner Temples and Inner Convocation is that they are *consubstantial loci*. Their continuity is perpetuated in two ways: the first is through shared creative imagery as described above, built and maintained through many centuries by human and spiritual interaction. The second is the resonant affinity that they bear to the fundamental cosmic forces, such as the Sevenfold Directions of Time, Space, and Movement. This affinity is shown in Figure Four, (The Sevenfold Directions).

The Inner Temples and their central hub at the Inner Convocation are more permanent than those outer temples that are, or were originally, built as vessels and physical outlets for their inner counterparts. The Inner Temples are known by many names and have many descriptions, but their functions continue beyond cultural definitions.

Such special constructs are really hyper-maps, enabling the spiritual energies of the enfolded and interleaved territories to be experienced in a more direct manner, even while we are still living within our limited outer-life of questing, mapping, and interaction. Many inner-plane constructs are maintained intentionally by their occupants: these are the familiar, or unfamiliar, halls, temples, territories associated with chosen spiritual paths. They are no more real than the confused map of the outer territories that we make to prevent ourselves from feeling lost, but when they are clear and consistent, their transparency allows a sense of the underlying territories to show through. Furthermore, the hyper-maps or Inner Temples help to keep us in balance during those moments of exalted and extended awareness when we experience the greater reality as a result of our spiritual practices. Most helpfully they also enable us to attune to those inner-plane contacts that live within them.

The Inner-Plane Contacts

In our allegory of the lost individual trying to map a territory, he/she interacts with others who also engaged in mapping. Sometimes they share maps, sometimes they fight over them. The manifest world, in which we think we live, can lead under certain circumstances to other territories: this is the key teaching of the Tree of Life. Within these other enfolded and interleaved territories there are many inhabitants. We evolve through our interactions, and typically these are interactions with other map-makers.

In the hyper-maps of the Inner Temple and Inner Convocation the map-makers are trans-human beings of evolved consciousness. More simply, they grew up a long time ago, and threw away the consensual maps that rigidify the mind, coming into a new condition of awareness that is not bound by outer time. Interaction with such trans-human beings is a core component of any spiritual tradition. A short exploration of the nature of such Inner Contacts is offered in Appendix Two.

As in alchemical so it is in spiritual transformation: the *materia* (ourselves) must be combined with other substances or subtle energies, to effect a transformation. Just as the metals were said to evolve deep within the Earth, affected by their Planetary powers and associated spiritual Emanations, reaching ultimately to the Stars and to the source of Being, so may we choose to evolve by a conscious participation in the same process. The hyper-map, though immensely valuable, is not enough, for our journey must also be energized and accelerated.

In Chapter Two, the hidden nature of telluric forces is discussed, including their relevance for humanity during this current time of profound change, and how relating to such forces in new ways can bring transformation.

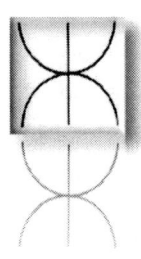

CHAPTER TWO

Working to Scale: Telluric Forces and the Human Imagination

Working to Scale

During the early months of 2010 and 2011 there were powerful earthquakes and huge storms. The planet vigorously reminded us of our human fragility: we are here only by the grace of the telluric underworld planetary forces that generate seismic movements and weather patterns. Within a short period, all too soon, we will forget our fragility and behave again as if we are the lords and masters of the world.

How does the impact of powerful planetary forces, within the Earth, affect our sacromagical work within the Sphere of Art? How may it affect our work with the earth-magic of the faery allies and the UnderWorld? And how does it affect our relationship to off-planet spiritual awareness, for the Sun and remote Stars are vast powers in themselves, far greater than our planet Earth. While we might have an idea or image of "the Sun" in meditation or vision, the margins for our safety, our very existence in the Solar field, are miniscule; somewhat closer and life on Earth burns, somewhat further off and life on Earth freezes. Solar activity may at any time negate our fragile electrical and communication networks, heralding a period of rapid and terrible collapse for modern civilization.

These are not wild doomsday prognostications; they are a simple statement of facts that we, as humans, are determined to ignore as we go on living, for there seems to be nothing we can do about them. No one forces us to live in earthquake zones, or on the slopes of volcanoes, but we continue to do so. No one gave any far-reaching thought to the location of nuclear power stations; they are equally dangerous wherever they are built. Yet we continue to build them, despite widespread concern about potential and actual disasters.

An uncomfortable truth for anyone doing sacromagical spiritual work of any kind is implied in the famous teaching of "as above, so below". If the physical Sun enables our life only within minute margins, how may we understand the spiritual Sun that is, so to speak, behind the physical entity? When we are withdrawn from that light we freeze and die within...this much is often attested in the spiritual traditions. Yet little is said about being burned through coming too close to the spiritual light.

The older traditions described hierarchies, lines of mediation, sets of images, through which the spiritual light and fire was gradually filtered. Regrettably this immensely valuable spiritual concept became progressively locked, stage by stage, into outer hierarchies of priest temples and churches, and the inner light withdrew from them. We might burn, or we might freeze. Today the individual must decide for his or her self how to come into a balanced relationship that cannot be hijacked. Fortunately there is help available, especially in the inner dimensions associated with spiritual evolution. Such help is not concerned with placing itself between us and the light as an authority, but with enabling us to come into communion with Being for ourselves. This is the purpose of the Inner Temples, mediated through the outer *Sanctuary of Avalon*, initiated by A. R. Heaver and Polly Wood in the 1950's, and continued by our Inner Temple members today in Glastonbury and the USA [7].

Telluric and Stellar Realities

If you have lived through an earthquake, a severe storm at sea, a volcanic eruption, a tsunami, your relationship to the telluric forces will have changed. No longer are they something that we try to "visualize" in our sacromagical work: they are more fully understood as the givers and takers of planetary life...all planetary life without exception. All life on Earth exists by the grace of the telluric powers, from the creatures of the air, to the largest on land or in sea, down to the microscopic life forms generated in the depths where volcanic fire meets the ocean waters. This is not a philosophical or metaphysical statement but factual, fully supported by modern science.

We may not remember, or even know, that the so-called solid earth beneath our feet is actually sliding around over raging telluric fires, but our state of innocence or willful ignorance does not imply that the inherent forces of our planet can be simply ignored, for we are influenced by them unceasingly. In this context of planetary forces the most powerfully *physical* is our much neglected, and oft-repudiated, gateway to the *spiritual*.

The Problem of Pseudo-knowledge

While our huge spiritual and magical revival, from the late 19th century to the present day has liberated many from the suppressive tyranny of authoritarian religion, it has also created an artificial comfort zone of false, or at best harmless and reassuring, pseudo- knowledge. The deeper esoteric traditions have been glossed over, in a process that has steadily created a new body of dogma no less restrictive than that of religion. This is most apparent in the New Age movement, but it is present also in revival witchcraft paganism and neo-shamanism, and in the current revival of practical magical arts. Signs of such dogma are most easily visible in the many boiler plate books on chakras, Wicca, and more recently neo-shamanism, repeating the basic material over and over, with little or no original research or development. While this may seem like trite harmless beginner's stuff at one level, it forms a rigid mass or crust of apparently unquestioned material that has accumulated during the last few decades. To challenge it often generates the kind of outrage that was once reserved for challenges to religious dogma. To accept it blindly is similar to submissively accepting religious dogma. The answer is never solely in books, though they may form an initial path toward answers, and few would deny that the right book, for some people, can be a powerful stimulus toward deeper spiritual exploration.

Our aim here is not to criticize, but to reveal deeper levels that may be worthy of meditation and dedicated sacromagical work.

After three generations or more of basic material within our overall magical/spiritual revival, material that has, in some streams, noticeably rigidified over the years, the time is right for further work and radical reassessment. Such a shake-up of received unchallenged material is similar to that of an earthquake...for a brief time all of our "knowns" and "givens" are shaken.

Forgetting Where We Are

Our comfortable forgetting of the true nature of our world is especially significant in sacromagical work with the deep earth forces. While, in scientific terms, there is little we can do if the mountain erupts, except flee, there are many significant implications and esoteric teachings regarding telluric forces, reaching at least as far back as the spiritual philosophy of Empedocles (circa 490-430 BCE). Yet almost all of this body of esoteric lore has been ignored and eventually forgotten. This absence of a major part of the esoteric tradition must be addressed, and in our Sphere of Art work, the foundation is first established by training in the UnderWorld and Faery Traditions, before moving on to any other aspects.

We Exist Within and Through the Seven Directions

Typically magical arts conceive of the Directions and the associated guardians/enablers, such as the Four Archangels, as being gateways to power: a ritual supposedly enhances and evokes energy. Ritualists repeatedly call upon the powers of the Directions, including the OverWorld and UnderWorld [8]. Modern reassessments of magical arts during the 20th and 21st centuries have brought UnderWorld and faery consciousness back into the picture after centuries of neglect and repudiation resulting from manipulative religious propaganda. Regrettably one of the crusts of the New Age is the sentimentalizing of both faeries and angels into trite product, and this is an area that requires rigorous attention.

Such essential reassessment is good, but it is by no means complete. There is still a great deal of UnderWorld spiritual work to explore, to reinstate, and most important of all, to move forward into the future. While we often start with ancestral wisdom, we must continue with a new wisdom that we forge from our own sacromagical and spiritual experience: that is what we, hopefully as wise ancestors, will ultimately leave to our heirs in the future.

Invocation, Evocation, and Power

In practice, and with experience, the popular ideas of "invocation and evocation", as employed today in practical magic, even by experienced and well-trained ritualists, must be called into question. Why? Because it seems more likely that the Guardians of the Directions have one main function: *to scale down and reduce the power*. If our invocations/evocations of the North, for example, were to have a telluric response, we might truly raise up mountains. If you have been in an earthquake or near an active volcano, you will know why such power is scaled *down* rather than *up* by the spiritual Guardians of the Directions during magical work, regardless of any cultural names or forms you may choose to give them. The words "angel" and "Archangel" are merely cultural and historical descriptive terms, not originative definitions, for the spiritual presences and powers exist regardless of our vocabulary.

Of course, we experience the process of scaling-down continually in our lives; it is part of the homeostatic balancing process whereby the planet corrects its energies and maintains equilibrium. Such equilibrium is a planetary function, not solely a human idea, and it is certainly not upon a human-supportive scale. A planetary equilibrium, especially the continuous correction process toward balance, does not take us into account, and we are almost irrelevant within it.

We happen to live briefly on a minute portion of the surface land. That surface land, as every school child knows, is but a small proportion of the watery ocean-dominated planetary surface.

We are minor, no matter what we think of ourselves, and that sums us up, in planetary terms. So much is discussed concerning our damaging effect upon the environment that we think of ourselves as paramount, but if we were to go, to become extinct, the Earth would regenerate very rapidly indeed in terms of planetary time. I do not make this statement about the vast potential for regeneration as any excuse for environmental crime; we are liable and responsible to tend, care for, and to love unfailingly our world, nothing less will suffice.

The sole and shocking exception to this regenerative potential is pollution from our nuclear generating plants and weapons, a terrible burden to leave for our descendants in exchange for the energy, and the culture, that drives our televisions, cell-phones, computers and entertainment simulacra.

Somehow, in the recent past of the last 2,000 years, we became enamored of the notion that we are somehow special, important, and the rulers of planet Earth. Where did this nonsense come from? Undoubtedly from a perspective rooted in the Book religions and their resultant materialism. Let us set it aside, and consider instead that our continued existence is entirely dependent upon that *scaling-down of power* mentioned above.

The scaling-down process that concerns us here is not just the planetary urge toward balance and homeostasis, but a minute mirroring of it, that mirroring which occurs in our sacromagical work, comparable in the most miniscule way to the macroscopic order of planetary homeostasis. To put it simply, if you try and "raise up power" and have any measure of success, there are potent and valid Guardian forces and entities, acting according to natural laws that will simply push it back down again: that is their sacred and enduring function. With this simple truth we discover the rift between the popular idea of magic, in which evocation and invocation of Power is much written about, but practiced with little effect, and a deeper sacromagical or theurgic perspective.

The Sphere of Art works to exclude certain forces rather than to evoke them. It is, paradoxically, a method of initially reducing energy rather than building it. The Guardians, typified as The Archangels (discussed later), seal and empty the Sphere: they do not pour "energy" into it according to human will, desire, or imagination. It only takes a few minutes of honest thought to grasp that there is absolutely no reason for Archangels, gods, goddesses, or planetary spirits, to empower humans: they have more significant acts to perform in the weaving and moving of the Earth, the Solar System, and the Cosmos. Can we truly stand, so to speak, in their beneficent light?

Only when we understand how protected, how beneficially limited we are, in our sacromagical work, can we begin to be truly effective. In the classic magical worldview, such wise limitation is often associated with the North, the cosmic Laws of Being, and the element of Earth. Such limitations associated with Earth require that to take *form* we must limit *force.* So if we were truly to invoke more than a minute degree of power, the first effect it would have, quite naturally and without any prejudice, would be to destroy us. This is the evident truth of the earthquake, the tidal wave, the volcanic eruption, the vast storm. There is no inherent "evil" in such arising powers, but their larger forces will frequently disrupt and destroy our smaller limited forms.

As it is in nature and in physics, so is it in super-nature and in metaphysics, with the proviso that the deeper wisdom of our outer sciences should always be informed by a spiritual perspective, rather than a materialistic greed and profit-driven agenda. Until we bring ethics completely to the foreground of science and medicine, we will continue to plummet down our path of self-destruction.

Energy, Form, and Consciousness

Up to this point we have discussed only energies and limitations, the seemingly infinite dialectic of force and form. We have not yet considered individual or group consciousness. Resonating between force and form is the consciousness that arises as a result of their interaction in the manifest world of Nature. This model of the interactive origin of consciousness is, significantly, shared by both materialistic and spiritual traditions, though each places a different emphasis upon the interaction. While the materialist perspective attempts to study the interactions through the brain and the body, the spiritual perspective suggests that brain and body are only outer organs, small parts of a bigger picture, and not the source, cause, or ultimate locations of consciousness.

In the metaphysical dimensions, the pattern of force and form interacting to generate consciousness takes a different shape, in which force and form arise as a *result* of consciousness, and not vice versa. Figure Five (Interaction of Force and Form) illustrates the model, and if you are familiar with the Tree of Life, you will immediately see certain connections. The universal consciousness, the Being from which all beings derive, emits the polarized patterns of force and form, and when they interact, they in turn emit a different mode of consciousness; that in which we live on Earth. This principle is often related to harmonics or overtones in music, which have long been employed as an acoustic physical demonstration of deeper laws of being.

The diagram shows the possibility of a through line from the greater consciousness (emitting or originating) to the lesser consciousness (interacting or expressing). This through line reaches into all entities in the manifest world of Nature, including ourselves. There is a pivotal point of interaction, marked (a), where force/form meet equally in consciousness from above and below. This could be conceived as deadlock or stasis, but in fact it is a point of vibrant balanced energy: a point of poise and potential.

How May We Use the Interaction Point?

The interaction point, or point of poise, is frequently sought in meditation: it can be accessed through Stillness practice. In many popular spiritual practices, there is a concept, often accepted without explanation or questioning, that our consciousness should, or must, *rise* toward its higher mode. It is difficult to avoid such terminology, and throughout this book I have attempted to show that it need not be the result of, or a cause for, divisive dualism. The answer is in practice, rather than in semantics.

This elevation, rising, presented in various ways according to cultural preference or spiritual traditions, moves the consciousness toward its source, that overtone or octave of consciousness that emits both force and form as expanding harmonics of its triad. In such movement upwards, we are often taught, we must *move away* from the manifesting consciousness in Nature that results from the interaction of force and form. This is the classic idea, much represented, little understood, of "rising through the planes" found in so many spiritual practices. Historically and psychologically it is based upon antagonistic dualism. The corollary, from which we daily suffer, is that the world and all within it is essentially product for our use and abuse. A more recent variant, widely promulgated, tells us that the good spiritual people will become enlightened, then "ascend", leaving the post-Christian materialists behind to play with their smartphones. Such a New Age dogma of escapist ascension is merely a fair-trade, hand-woven, artisan cover for the stark medieval Christian belief in salvation of the few with damnation for the rest. This cruel and manipulative propaganda continues to permeate religious fundamentalism today.

While such rising through the planes is indeed possible and often remarkable, it has implications that are often ignored or intentionally glossed over. As we move beyond that interaction point (a) and toward the originating consciousness, we lose the dynamic of force and form. Indeed, this loss is regarded as a valuable end in itself in many spiritual traditions...losing the interplay of energy and substance, force and form. It is, for example, the openly hidden key to releasing *karma* as understood within popularized Eastern philosophy.

Through the Sphere of Art and the telluric spiritual forces, we invite or allow, but not command, the Rising Light from the planet to give us a push or boost. This Rising Light moves us beyond the interaction point (a), but it comes from *beneath* the consciousness in Nature, as shown in our Figure Six (The Rising Earth Light). Thus the impetus to rise Above or off-planet comes from Below or in-planet and we *ride upon it*.

For those familiar with the Jewish Merkavah (Markava, Merkabah) tradition of Kabbalistic mysticism, as distinct from the various solipsistic New Age presentations that cannot be commented upon in detail here, this concept reveals something that is usually hidden. While Markava mysticism describes rising through the planes, halls, or metaphysical dimensions, the practice itself is called *descending* through the Markava [9].

Riding the Chariot, Uplifting the World

In sacromagical work of this sort, our practice with the Sphere gradually builds for us an energetic vessel, in ancestral cultures called a Chariot. Such terminology is handed down to us from an era when the chariot was the most rapid mode of transport.

We could also call it the Vehicle. This Vehicle is built from our own energies of interaction, force-form-consciousness, attuned in a new and more effective manner than that of habituated daily life. Variants of this practice are found in spiritual or sacromagical traditions from many cultural sources, ancient and contemporary. The significant difference in our Sphere of Art method is that telluric or UnderWorld energy must be ridden carefully, like skillful balancing upon a powerful rising tide, and that the inherent movement is not dependent upon the will or whim of the rider, but comes from within the sacred planet which is a boundless source of spiritual transformation.

It follows that such tidal forces or expanding energies are also present from the Moon, Sun, and Planets, but whereas we are receptive to those that seem to come "from above" we can participate directly in the rising Earth Light "from below". Typically we are unconscious of all of this, though popular astrology gives some limited insights through the natal and progressed chart of the individual.

When we move consciousness in the manner described above, allowing the Earth Light to lift or push us from below, as distinct from the typical "rising through the planes" method that almost inevitably involves escape, we maintain some intentional connection with that natural interaction of force and form, of polarity of energies. We do not lose our contact with the world of Nature, but instead it first initiates movement as it uplifts us, then it is *uplifted with us*. This effect is most apparent within our own consciousness, manifesting through the physical body, but also resonates to our surrounding environment.

If a substantial number of people consciously worked with the rising Earth Light in this manner, the planet would be transformed.

The Four Guardians or Archangels

As described above, there is much confusion over the function and nature of the Archangels, and many prohibitions regarding interaction with them. As always with prohibitions, we have to explore what the prohibition conceals. It seems odd, to say the least, that tables of Archangels were published in previous centuries, and noted by hand in early Kabbalistic schools, along with strict rules about never working with them! This curious habit found its way into publication, of course, and into many ostensibly Christian mystical magical or alchemical sources. It has often been interpreted, with some justification, as an injunction against the corrupting influence of potential polytheism, at least as far as monotheism is concerned. Yet the prohibition, combined with detailed revelation, is really an injunction for the initiate: do not work with them lightly or in superstitious worship, but seek to understand them and work with them wisely.

In our source text of *Aesch Mezareph, the Purifying Fire,* no reference is made to Archangels or angels. In our Sphere of Art practice, we bring them back into the field.

The Sphere of Art is first emptied and sealed by the Guardians, typified as the Four Archangels, *Raphael, Michael, Gabriel,* and *Auriel*. These Archangels were originally, and still are, the planetary intelligences associated with Mercury, Sun, Moon, and Venus, mediating spiritual forces of Brilliance, Harmony, Foundation, and Exaltation. Before they were called "Archangels" they had other names, but their functions were the same then as now, often beyond our simple human interpretation of Solar and Lunar time cycles. We may give such beings many names, many descriptions, many cultural attributions, but they are not changed much thereby. Only their *interface* with us will change according to our cultural background. The words *angel* and *Archangel* are from Greek, while the concept and much of the potent imagery found in tradition, come from Assyrian or Babylonian tradition, absorbed by Jewish culture and religion, later to permeate into Christianity and Islam.

Planetary Intelligences Defined

What, therefore, is a "planetary intelligence?" From an exoteric perspective, the concept of planetary intelligences is found in myth and legend from ancient cultures. It can vary from folk tales to sophisticated temple traditions. In all such examples, the movement and influence of a celestial body is given a persona, an interface that somehow describes or attempts to explain not only physical celestial movements and rhythms, but traditional associations of power, function, role, interaction, and so forth. From such a basis, found in sacromagical and mythic lore worldwide, comes the familiar idea of the pantheon of gods and goddesses associated with the Sun Moon and Planets.

Over time, and through various cultural and religious changes, the spiritual traditions of Judaism and Christianity took unto themselves certain ancient attributes of planetary intelligences, especially those of ancient Persia. Early Islam also adopted these traditions, and sophisticated metaphysics relating to spiritual consciousness and planetary intelligences is found in both Jewish and Islamic Qabalah [10] both containing complex Zoroastrian influences. Both streams repeatedly assert that the Planets are not, in themselves, deities or spirits. They stand, in the material cosmos, as manifest signs for deeper forces of creation destruction and harmony, but are not the forces themselves.

Much of this complex metaphysics can be simplified into one statement acceptable to both modern physics and to metaphysics: the *entities of the Solar System mediate energy to one another, out of and into the cosmos.* This creates a powerful meditation, and is deeply rooted in the hidden methods of Qabalah, whereby a direct relationship is developed, rather than one replete with images or symbols [11].

How we may describe that energy, traditionally embodied in Archangels and angels, and studied by modern physics, where it comes from, where it goes, how we react to it, is found in the various models of "reality" that range from hard-line materialistic science and quantum mechanics to abstruse esoteric teachings.

The Guardians, Archangels, or messengers are beings of consciousness and energy. They mediate forces exchanged between the physical entities of the Solar System and beyond. While the entities are physical, as Moon, Sun, Planets and Stars, the energies extend into their original source of the Tenfold Emanations, shown upon the Tree of Life, pre-existing in metaphysical dimensions.

In the Western esoteric tradition four main guardians, Archangels, or messengers have long been established as having a special relationship to humanity, by which we should also understand, to planet Earth. Over time their role has been progressively downplayed in exoteric religion, but esoterically their significance has continued for many centuries, reaching back to their earlier origins with different names and different cultural attributes. Ultimately we become aware of them in meditation and theurgic ritual: from that stage onwards we discover their true names, which are the unique identifying subtle forces that they convey.

The Significance and Function of the Four Archangels

The associations of the Four Guardians or Four Archangels with the Moon, Mercury, Venus, and the Sun, are frequently confused or contradictory in publication, and there are many tangled motifs in their representation in religious and sacromagical iconography. Rather than list the variations, as has been done repeatedly, perhaps we should first ask: why are these Four Guardians of special significance?

On the standard Tree of Life, shown in Figure Seven (Archangels upon the Tree), they can be seen as the first four entities and powers encountered on *ascending* from Earth, or conversely, as the most powerful entities or forces *descending* into the Earth, as they receive the forces of all the other Emanations, then combine them together into the Foundation and Kingdom, through the manifest forms of our Moon and Earth. Ascending and descending are relative terms, from our gravity-bound perspective. In fact they neither ascend nor descend, but radiate permeate and move toward and away from our planet in all directions.

A helpful meditation is one in which we steadily replace Up and Down from planet Earth with Within and Without...movement to and from the center. Such movement is spherical and simultaneous in all directions, but we habitually isolate part of it relative to ourselves upon the planetary surface and subject to gravity.

The physical entities of Moon, Mercury, Venus, Sun, in ascending order on the Tree of Life, are nodes or ingress-points for greater energies coming into our planet from the galaxy, from the cosmos. In other words, the physical entities are also mediating entities. Likewise, they are the nodes or egress-points for energies moving from our planet into the Solar System and cosmos. This interaction was traditionally understood as a Conversation between the Earth and the Solar System. It is the origin of the significant metaphysical model representing the Music of the Spheres, and of much ancient astrology.

By working with the Four Archangels, through the laws of harmonics, we are already working with the deeper forces embodied by Mars, Jupiter, Saturn, Neptune, and Uranus, as is shown on the Tree of Life. This harmonic relationship is not limited to the classic astrological model alone, but should be understood upon the Tree of Life as including those astrological attributes subsumed within a greater set, such as the originating Ten Emanations and their spiritual powers.

Here we should note that the classic astrological attributes are most recognizable when an individual lives within the reactive consciousness of Nature, that is, within a web of consciousness arising from that manifest interaction of force and form described above and shown in our Figure Five. If he or she intentionally moves awareness though consistent spiritual practice and discipline toward the next point, (a) in Figure Five, the *overtones* of the astrological attributes come into effect, and the natal chart may be re-formed and activated in a new way.

Another helpful model describing this transformation is that of Figure Eight (The Three Wheels), whereby the individual who consciously moves into the point of poise has moved from within the repetitions or cycles of the Wheel of Fortune, into the balancing of force and form, creation and destruction, Mercy and Severity, of the Wheel of Justice. The greater Wisdom and Understanding, beyond and behind our many lifetimes, is that of the Wheel of Judgment.

UnderWorld Considerations

According to the perennial spiritual traditions, the basis of all Alchemy, the planetary forces of the Solar System are found also within the body of our Earth, as the metals and elements, the substances described in alchemical tradition; hence the close connection between the Planets, the Metals, and other primary substances such as Sulphur Salt and Mercury. We find this connection still developing today, whereby new elements found in the Earth (embodying UnderWorld forces) are still given mythic planetary names by materialist science, plutonium and uranium being the best known of a long list, many of them more recent.

Such mirroring of the forces of the Solar System as metallic and elemental forms within the Earth, according to perennial spiritual and sacromagical traditions, has much to offer us in our quest for deeper understanding. Just as the powerful telluric forces of earthquake, volcano, and storm physically embody spiritual energies of transformation, so do the metals and elements. Such embodiment is not a matter of comparison intellectual or factual relationship alone, but one of interaction and transformation. It is through such interaction and transformation that we live, and it may be both accelerated and purified in spiritual alchemical terminology through our *conscious participation* in the processes of change. This process is none other than that of *Aesch Mezareph*.

Alchemy proposes and describes a mysterious evolution of the metals from lead to gold that is said to occur naturally within the planetary body, but may, under controlled circumstances, be replicated in a sealed vessel. Such controlled circumstances are often described in ways that imply a fusion of subtle forces and catalytic reactions. We must have both for the metals to evolve or transmute.

This same process is possible within our consciousness and energy. The Sphere of Art creates in miniature the interactions of *Aesch Mezareph*, the Purifying Fire within the body of the planet. Due to the metals and minerals within our body, we can initiate our own transformation through methods associated with the vessel or Sphere, the Fire of Transformation, and the Rising Light from the planetary heart.

The Archangels and the Metals

The Four Guardians/Archangels have a special resonance with celestial and telluric entities and energies, with forms and forces. Such associations are well known, in ascending order, as :

Silver/Moon/Gabriel;

Mercury/Mercury/Raphael;

Copper/Venus/Auriel;

Gold/Sun/Michael.

These metals are vital to our health and consciousness, yet are poisonous in anything more than minute amounts. *Thus our reaction to the metals found in the Earth restates, and mirrors in miniature, the limiting power of the Guardians on a greater scale.*

Just as the telluric forces of the planetary plates are contained and held in balance for what are short periods of time in terms of planetary lifetime (though long indeed to us), so are the destructive forces of the sacred metals. Through such containment they become beneficial, providing we understand how to work with them. This is the great secret of Alchemy. The same principle is found in homeopathy, whereby minute doses of substances that cause illness or imbalance can be taken to generate a wholesome re-balancing through stimulating the vital forces needed for recovery.

Gold and Silver are given especial value by humans as "wealth", originally due to their mediation of Solar and Lunar forces. We can see only too clearly how obsession with "wealth" as an abstract artificially enforceable power has brought our culture to the point of collapse in the early 21st century.

In addition to the primary associations of the Four Archangels, we have further sets arising from their mediation of higher planetary spheres and emanations. This is shown on the Tree of Life, in Figure Eight (The Three Wheels).

The Four Archangels in Sequence, from Earth to Sun

Look up at the sky: the nearest and most rapidly moving body is the Moon. Then come Mercury and Venus, so visible to our ancestors at dawn and dusk, and during the day the vast entity of the Sun. We can explore each of the Four Guardians or Archangels in sequence, starting with the one closest to us.

Gabriel (silver/Moon) *adapts* and *modifies* energies of the Sun/gold by *reflection.* Likewise there is a further adaptation and modification of stellar energies both via the Sun, as a Star, and through faint but all –pervading stellar forces acting directly upon the Moon and in the Sub-Lunar realm between Moon and Earth. Significantly for our era, the First Emanation, or Crown of the Tree, has been associated in our time with Uranus. Thus Gabriel acts an *isklaria* or mirror for the forces of Michael, Archangel of the Sun, and of Metatron, Archangel of the Throne or Crown. Metatron is the Archangel that contains all others: the Archangels of the Tree of Life are all organs of Metatron.

Gabriel primarily works through Silver, but has a subtle influence through gold and uranium. Uranium is, for us on Earth, an UnderWorld element, reminding us of the teaching that the Kingdom of Earth is simultaneously the Crown of the Stellar Heavens, but "after another manner". This refers to the law of octaves: a more simple description might be that planet Earth and the Stars have something in common with one another at their deepest core of Being. In more recent years Pluto/plutonium has been associated with the middle pillar of the Tree of Life, at the Crossing from the Solar realm to the trans-Solar or Stellar realms (Figure One). Thus Gabriel can mediate uranium/Uranus, plutonium/Pluto, gold/Sun, through its primary metal of silver. There is a significant meditation in this sequence, which comprises the Middle Pillar or Axis Mundi.

We will discover that Gabriel is associated with other UnderWorld elements or metals, when we consider the UnderWorld Tree.

Gabriel also modulates, through the Moon, the forces of Mercury/mercury and Venus/copper. As the harmonic metals and spiritual powers of Sun, Venus, Mercury, all mediate the forces of Mars, Jupiter, Saturn, Uranus, and Pluto, we can meditate on the potency of Gabriel that brings the entire Tree of Life in modulated form through the Lunar realm, to life on Earth. This mediation of Emanations through Sun, Venus, Mercury, and Moon, is shown on the standard Tree of Life, which is, in part, a map of our relativistic observation of the Solar System from the surface of planet Earth.

While Gabriel and the Lunar realm are often described as "lower" it could be argued, from the evidence above, that Gabriel is the most powerful of the Archangels for us, here on Earth. Traditionally, the Four Archangels are interpreted as having equal powers, but different interacting functions.

The Sub-Lunar World

The old term for our world was the Sub-Lunar World. This definition is well worth meditation and deeper exploration, for it truly describes where and how we live. The Sub-Lunar world is the zone of interaction, at all levels of being and energy, comprising Earth and Moon, together. The Moon weaves a sphere around the Earth, orbiting rapidly day and night. Everything within that sphere is Sub-Lunar, and we could further meditate that we are living within the sphere of the Moon. It is in this sense that we find the oft- written magical idea of the Moon, Foundation, as being just before form, and a subtle sea of malleable fertility both biologically and in consciousness. This Sub-Lunar realm, sphere of the Moon, is the constantly manifesting aspect of the Foundation, or 9th Emanation.

Modern physics has discovered that both Earth and Moon orbit around a locus or barycenter within the body of the Earth. They are two poles of one entity. Curiously, we find a similar model in metaphysics surviving up to and beyond the Renaissance period, but gradually fading out in occult texts from the 18th and 19th centuries onwards. By the 20th century, Moon and Earth have frequently become separated in esoteric literature and, as a result, in spiritual practice. The Moon has become limited as a realm of dreams and the unconscious mind due to the influence of materialist psychology, yet the dream and supposedly unconscious modes are only a small part of the Sub-Lunar world.

The dual entity of Earth and Moon together is the Foundation referred to in perennial philosophy or Qabalah: "The Earth, firmly Founded and not lightly moved" as it is described in the 12th century *Vita Merlini* [3]. The Kingdom, often used to refer to Earth only, should be understood as all manifest expressed form throughout the cosmos. Our planet is, of course, that aspect of the Kingdom best known to us, within which we have our being. The universal Kingdom, and the universal Foundation, with their ceaseless interaction, are each mirrored by our dual-entity of Earth and Moon. This same reflection is found within us, and is the openly hidden key to most practical magical work.

Raphael (Mercury/quicksilver-mercury). Raphael mediates and modulates the energies of the Sun/gold, Venus/copper, and Mars/iron, in addition to the primary metal of quicksilver. Overtones are those of Saturn/lead. Note that the *overtone* is a metal associated with *underworld* telluric forces, as lead contains and protects against the effects of radiation from x-rays, and heavy metals such as uranium and plutonium.

Auriel (Venus/copper) also mediates and modulates energies of the Sun/gold, Mercury/quicksilver. The primary mediation, however, is that of Jupiter/tin, with its higher octave of Neptune/salt.

Michael (Sun/gold) is the one Archangel of the four that would seem to have no direct path to Earth. Its power is mediated and modulated through the Moon, Mercury, and Venus. Michael is associated harmonically with Mars/iron, Jupiter/, Saturn/lead, Neptune/salt and Pluto/plutonium and Uranus/uranium or traditionally crystalline sulphur, as the Paths of Connection all center on the 6th Emanation of the Sun, Harmony, and Beauty.

Archangels and Gender

Michael is associated with the Sun. When we discuss Archangels, "it" is the correct term, rather than "he", as Archangels are always before and beyond gender. (Although "it" is often considered pejorative in modern use when referring to a living person, "it" originally was used in English as descriptive of a third gender or pre-sexual state; children before puberty were called "it". Nowadays "it" refers mainly to inanimate objects, hence its accumulated but inaccurate pejorative use when describing a person).

Michael is traditionally described as the Solar Archangel. When we use the term "he" freely, our relationship to the Archangel is essentially receptive, therefore its power is outgoing and stereotypically "masculine" to us. However, maintaining a good and strong contact with Archangels substantially depends on our image of them: trite religious or New Age sentimental images of angels and Archangels will only put us into contact with trite and sentimental spirit beings, claiming to be what we seek, but often masquerading, and of a lesser nature.

Archangels are androgynous; their state of being is before gender. There is much to be discovered by reversing the accepted gender-roles of Archangels and meditating upon them as feminine...something that is seldom done due to religious stereotyping and centuries of conditioning.

The Gender Meditation

Then lifted I up mine eyes, and looked, and, behold, there came out two women, and the wind was in their wings; for they had wings like the wings of a stork. Zachariah 5:9

Meditation: A powerful exercise is to meditate upon a specific Archangel as masculine and feminine in turn. What are the differences, how do they feel?

If masculine and feminine are the first two stages of a meditational practice, the third stage is to conceive of, and meditate upon, and steadily come into communion with, the Archangel as androgynous: this is the most powerful. One method is to envision the masculine and feminine aspects and energies as right and left radiant emissions from the Archangel, then to follow them to the source, where they merge. This is the origin of an old visionary method, whereby streams of angels are envisioned flowing out of and into their originating Archangel. The source, the true nature of the Archangel, is always a condition before the polarization that we call gender.

This exercise is valuable to human consciousness, especially toward liberation of stereotypes within us, but it is entirely about our inner responses, and does not affect the Archangels themselves in any way. They can be feminine, masculine, or androgynous, or even another gender altogether, depending on our approach to them and our reception of them.

While there is a mutual polar relationship between us and the angelic/Archangelic beings, it is not gender specific, but is about exchange of subtle energies. As mentioned above, our main experience of Archangels is receptive, just as our main experience of the Sun Moon Planets and Stars is receptive: here on Earth we receive these vast energies, modified through their mutual interaction, and especially modified by Lunar influence.

The Archangelic Cycle of the Elements

We often identify angels and Archangels through anthropomorphized images of the mobile active forces of the cosmos, embodying *formless power* into a concrete shape or presentation for the human consciousness. When this formless power touches the Elements, like a ray or beam, they are stirred thereby, and resolve into new forms. Each Archangel or angel carries or declares the power of one main Element, thus they will interact strongly with their native Element, but also with the other three. This is the key to a wide range of sacromagical practices. A classic meditation is to attune to one of the Archangels, and perceive and commune with it through each of the Elements in turn, beginning with its polar opposite Element, and ending with its own strong Element. Thus for Michael, we would begin with Earth and end with Fire. A simple table demonstrates this meditational cycle:

Raphael: through Water, Earth, Fire, and **Air**.

Michael: through Earth, Water, Air, **Fire**.

Gabriel: through Air, Fire, Earth, **Water**.

Auriel: through Fire, Water, Air, **Earth**.

In each of these forms, the order of the middle two elements of the series can be exchanged. Thus we can build a second cycle as follows:

Raphael: through Water, Fire, Earth, and **Air**.

Michael: through Earth, Air, Water, and **Fire**.

Gabriel: through Air, Earth, Fire, **Water**.

Auriel: through Fire, Air, Water, **Earth**.

The two cycles will provide some simple meditative Sigils, as shown in Figure Twenty Two, (The Sigils of the Archangels and Elements).

Michael rules the radiant outpouring light and fire energies of the Sun. In tradition, this Archangel and its component hosts of angels, the 6th Order called *Malakhim*, act as Movement, Radiance, and Connection. So it is not a deity of the Sun, but the awareness within, and power of, a vast energetic *movement* of light, fire, and balance that holds the wheel of the Solar System together. The word *Malakh* is often translated as messenger though this is a general term for all angels: they are all Messengers. *Malakhim* (plural) also means spokes...as in spokes of a chariot wheel.

Many of the cautions in traditional Qabalah are against relating to spiritual forces, including angels and Archangels, as if they are deities. In Jewish tradition, of course, this derives from the concern over potential reversions to paganism or threats to monotheism, thought to be inherent within many long-established spiritual and magical practices. At a deeper level of understanding, the same principles can hold good. We do not worship angels and Archangels as deities, but not for dogmatic reasons; *to conceive of them as gods or goddesses would be to lose our proper relationship to them*. If we lose this relationship, we lose many opportunities for transformation and spiritual evolution.

Telesms of Power in Action

Here on Earth, Michael becomes the image for all that is in balance, and mediates energy of radiance and protection, that shining force within which our world bathes and moves, hence the traditional associations with noon, mid-summer, elemental fire, and physical and spiritual light.

Michael is not a god of light, and not the Solar Being itself, but the Radiant Utterance, Movement, and Integrity of that being. We might consider all Archangels as power in action, but not as the original sources that utter forth the power. Yet to us, each Archangel can and does appear to be highly "personified" in tradition.

This personification, of Michael and all angels or Archangels, is due to the building of *telesms* over thousands of years, in many traditions. Such telesms are established thought-forms and iconic images that mediate the raw power in a humanized mode, in response to ritual, known prayers and invocations, meditation and contemplation. They will also respond to *mediation* (as distinct from meditation) in ritual, something that we focus on in our Inner Temple methods.

In the Sanctuary of Avalon [7] specific Archangelic forces are mediated not just by trained human participants, but by powerful and enduring inner spiritual contacts associated with the inner stellar Fire Temple.

Michael is one of the forces used in certain key transformations of energy and consciousness. It works especially with the neck and spine, and the Rod in ritual magic. A Rod, a spine, is also a *Malakh* the straight yet flexible that connects and enables movement, somewhat like a spoke of a chariot wheel, that must strengthen, support, hold at a distance, yet flex gently as necessary without collapsing.

Archangels as Mirrors and Lenses

Another way of describing the function of an angel or Archangel, in traditional sacromagical or spiritual terminology, is that they *stand before*. An angel stands before an *aspect* of divine Being. Thus it is a lens through which the "light" of a divine aspect passes. When light passes through a lens it is modified or focused according to the design of that lens, and this is exactly what angels and Archangels do: they stand before any aspect of Divine Being, and modulate its power according to their nature. We could regard each as a lens of differing shape and facets, yet the same light passes through each, and thus they modulate spiritual consciousness and power.

In traditional Qabalah all angels/Archangels upon the Tree of Life are organs of a greater over-being, called Metatron.

Metatron stands before the Throne of the Crown, mediating the Being that utters all beings in all worlds. The consciousness and energy of the angels/Archangels are also reflected, mirrored, in the human body, based upon the interactions shown upon the Tree of Life.

The Sequence of the Archangels from Earth to Stars

10 Sandalphon: feet/Earth. Kingdom of manifestation

9 Gabriel: genitals (vessel of hips and loins) /Moon. Foundation of form.

8 Raphael: right side of body/Mercury. Honor, Glory, Scintillation, Thought (left hemisphere).

7 Auriel: left side of body/Venus. Victory, Power, Exaltation, Emotion (right hemisphere).

6 Michael: heart (vessel of heart and lungs)/Sun. Beauty, Harmony, central Will.

5 Khamiel: right arm and hand of power/Mars. Severity, Discipline, Purification.

4 Tzadkiel: left arm and hand of peace/Jupiter. Mercy, Expansion, Compassion.

3 Tzaphkiel: right shoulder and right side of face/Saturn. Understanding, Inclusion.

2 Ratziel: left shoulder and left side of face/Neptune. Wisdom, Declaration.

1/10 Metatron: entire face and head (vessel of whole body)/Uranus. Crown of Spirit.

The Three Vessels

The Lunar and Solar entities each form a center, the locus or core of a Vessel. Thus the Lunar Vessel receives Sun, Venus, Mercury, and the higher octaves of Stars, Uranus, Saturn, Pluto, and Neptune. This Lunar Vessel receives and blends the modulated forces of all the higher Emanations, before they pass to Earth. As we have seen above, the Emanations embodied by Mercury and Venus can act directly upon Earth, and further mediate the higher overtones of Mars and Saturn (Mercury), and Jupiter and Neptune (Venus).

The Solar Vessel receives Mars, Jupiter, Pluto, Saturn, Neptune, and Uranus. As we have seen above, Mercury and Venus can also act directly upon the Sub-Lunar Realm.

Tradition and experience both reveal that our Earth is a receiving Vessel of all the Emanations, thus giving us Three Vessels, shown in Figure Nine.

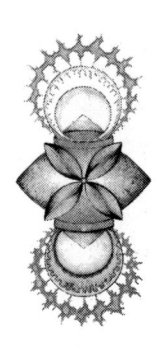

In Chapter Three we will discover how to apply these ancient traditional concepts in practical transformation within the Sphere of Art. As is often the case, that which seems complex on paper is simple in practice, and with some patient repetition, the transformations within the Sphere of Art will open out rapidly.

CHAPTER THREE

Working with the Metals and Minerals

The traditional metals, minerals, and substances for *Aesch Mezareph* are well-defined in our source text and in many other sources on Alchemy and Qabalah There are however variations, blinds, Qabalistic references (including puns and jokes) that are often intended to confuse students, or at least challenge them to think for themselves. In the 19th century edition of *Aesch Mezareph* by Dr. Wynn Westcott, available on-line or in facsimile editions, the editor states explicitly that the order of relationship of metals to the Emanations of the Tree of Life, as mediated by the Planets, has been intentionally confused in the original text. Some of his observations are quoted in Chapter Seven, and in the Appendices and End Notes

This intentional confusion was standard practice, and older texts were always intended for an oral elucidation, during long periods of testing and refining in both spiritual and physical work. Nowadays we no longer need such a testing-by-confusion approach, especially as the correct alignments of the Tree of Life and the metals are well known and extensively published. Furthermore, we must gently and positively adapt for the times in which have chosen to live; it is better by far to have a good clean start, with obfuscation cleared away [11].

The Dry Way and the Wet Way

Traditional Alchemy frequently referred to two paths: The Dry Way, and the Wet Way. These paths are interpreted in many different manners, and presented through many variants in literature. There is no claim, or even a suggestion, that the methods in this book are the only or true techniques. But if you work with these methods steadily as described, you will experience transformative results and many deep insights as your consciousness is clarified beyond the consensual and individual maps.

Both of the traditional paths are followed within the Sphere of Art, beginning with the Dry Way. In some alchemical sources the Dry Way is considered to be a potentially dangerous shortened-way process, though we must allow for some typical flamboyance and mystique when we read such accounts. As a true caution this may refer to strong chemical/alchemical reactions that can occur, if the hidden method is not faithfully followed. The causes of such reactions are bypassed in our method of the Dry Way, and are not, therefore, a potential risk.

As stated above, there are many variants in literature and in practice. The inexperienced student is often baffled and frustrated by this, and the materialist shrugs it all off as nonsense. The true answer, the true materials, and the true method, are as follows: choose a path and follow it faithfully without digression to its end. When you have done this, all paths will become clear to you, and confusion will have ceased.

Our method for use in the Sphere of Art is partly derived from perennial tradition, and the foundation of the *Aesch Mezareph* text, but it offers a unique and previously unpublished way of working. The techniques are supported by teachings from my mentors, and communication and inspiration from Inner Contacts, those advanced trans-human beings met in the Inner Temples, and associated with the ancient sacromagical tradition behind the Sanctuary of Avalon. However, there is no requirement for you to "believe" in any of this source material, as faith plays no part in the process. If you try it, follow it carefully through its few simple stages, you will feel it work within you. The rest is commentary.

The Metals and Substances Defined

Even a brief survey of alchemical texts will show that the range of substances employed is ordered according to metal, mineral, animal, and vegetable. Within the Sphere of Art we will be working primarily with the metals and the mineral world. For practical work the primary substances may be embodied as follows:

10th Emanation, expressed in the Solar System by Earth: Carbon or Lava. *The Kingdom of Manifestation.*

9th Emanation, expressed in the Solar System by Moon: *Silver. The Foundation.*

8th Emanation, expressed by Mercury: *Quicksilver (Mercury). Glory or Scintillation.*

7th Emanation, expressed by Venus: *Copper. Victory or Exaltation.*

6th Emanation, expressed by the Sun: Gold. *Beauty, Harmony, Balance.*

5th Emanation, expressed by Mars: Iron. *Severity, Rigor, Purification.*

4th Emanation, expressed by Jupiter: Tin. *Mercy, Bounty, Compassion.*

3rd Emanation, expressed by Saturn: Lead. *Understanding.*

2nd Emanation, expressed by Neptune: Natural Sea Salt. *Wisdom.*

1st Emanation, expressed by Uranus: *Crystal (Quartz or Sulphur). Crown.*

While the Planets mediate and express the spiritual transcendent Emanations in the Heavens, the substances directly embody their spiritual forces within planet Earth.

Sulfur, Salt, and Mercury

Although crystal is referred to, in this method, we by-pass most contemporary or New Age material regarding crystals: we are working in a different manner. Traditionally crystalline Sulphur represents Life and Spirit, while crystalline Salt is Spirit as Substance. Sulphur is the higher octave as Spirit and Life in the 1st Emanation, the Crown, while Salt is the manifest octave in essential substance, through evaporation, the Kingdom. We always consider Salt to be the product of *Wisdom*, associated with the 2nd Emanation, but for us, wisdom through experience...

a metaphor that has often been employed. Sulfur and Salt each have a higher octave and a lower, the higher overtone in the Supernal Emanations, and the lower manifest on Earth. The Salt for your practical work must be a natural untreated sea salt. In a metaphysical context, Salt stands for all salts, and Sulphur stands for all crystals.

Mercury, which is mysteriously both liquid and metal, was traditionally understood to be the flow or link between Above, Spirit, Sulfur, and Below, Body, Salt. In Alchemy the terms Sulfur Mercury and Salt often mean qualities or conditions, (as in *like unto* sulfur, salt, mercury) and are not limited to the manifest substances described by those names.

Sulfur, with its inclination to Fire and Air, and Salt, with its inclination to Water and Earth, are also descriptive terms for sulfur-like action and salt-like action. Mercury, with its flowing ambiguous nature, is whatever flows between substances or elements in action, enabling transformation.

In a simple sense, Mercury is the Messenger: ever moving between Who and What, Above and Below. These three, Sulfur, Salt, and Mercury, are the primary triad of alchemical qualities, and of relative terminology.

In our Sphere of Art work we bypass much of the terminology, while honoring its inner meaning and content. So when we say "Sulfur" "Salt" and "Mercury" we mean that the substances of those names, found in nature, are our actual starting point and materials. We typically do not use the terms allegorically, but must nevertheless be aware of the higher octaves of all ten substances, through meditation and Sphere of Art work.

We have all of the substances listed above in minute amounts in our bodies, through the fluids, cells, right down to crystalline particles in our deepest bones. They exist in varying proportions within the primary qualitative roots of Air, Fire, Water, and Earth. Remember that all Four Roots or Elements are present varying proportions in each or any substance, and in each Emanation.

Some substances are qualitatively or relatively more resonant of certain Elements and less of others; as mentioned above, sulfur is of Fire and Air, salt of Water and Earth. This elemental understanding is still widespread in popular speech, perhaps the last active remnant of Element typology in modern consciousness: we hear someone described as fiery, earthy, an air-head, watery, and flavors are still given Elemental labels, such as those on bottles of wine.

The Elemental Cycle of Transformation

Interaction is the basis of the Elements and Triplicities [38] in astrology, and in traditional metaphysics magic and Alchemy, as in Figure Ten, (The Triplicities). For our purposes we apply this model, and that of the Three Wheels, to elicit transformation. Typically, but not exclusively, the stages are as follows:

1: **The Wheel of Fortune.** There is a natural process of transformation within the body that occurs through the diurnal and seasonal cycles of nature. It tends in all cases to follow the Wheel of Fortune, as shown in the classic Tarot trump of the same name, or the Cycle of the Elements. From Beginning to Completion, Birth to Death, Spring to Winter, Youth to Age, Dawn to Dusk, Air to Earth, and so forth, as shown in Figure Eleven (The Wheel of Life).

When this cycle is imbalanced the individual can become "ill" physically, mentally/emotionally, or be inhibited by a spiritual malaise. This might be exemplified by the cycle shuddering, slowing, or having a stop-start pattern. To become "well" we seek to restore the cycle to its smooth rotation, finally coming to rest at the point of death. In a normal life cycle there is no thought of suspending the rotation of the wheel or of working with it consciously. Such conscious acts may require specialized theurgic, thaumaturgical or sacromagical activities.

2: **Element of Earth.** The fourfold cycle may be accelerated or *catalyzed* through the minimal addition of chosen physical substances/energies that initiate change. Such changes may at first be therapeutic, then in the later stages are spiritually transformative. We might also say that they are immediately spiritually transformative, and that this initiation of spiritual forces can work its way progressively through into the physical body.

The difference between, and the relationship of, these effects derives from the influence of the Evolutionary and Involutionary streams, the Red and White Dragons. It is all a matter of movement and direction.

Thus far the transformation can be unconscious, and this is how most life patterns work. Typically, but not exclusively, the unconscious transformation is when the spiritual forces make steady changes through into the physical body. This is, as we all know, the cycle from birth to death, from innocence to experience, from ignorance to wisdom. It is replicated in miniature in any healing or transformative cycle. There are often examples whereby the spiritual forces are inhibited, and can cause dramatic sudden change, such as shocking events that undo the rigidity of the Self. The more rigid we are, the more inflexibly we hold on to our map and refuse to address the territory around us, the more likely we are to experience shocks. If we are open to change, we adapt to it more readily.

Conscious transformation is typically, but not exclusively, from the physical toward the spiritual. It is demonstrated by the well-known phrase "working on ones' self" though there are many illusions of what such work may be along the way. Thus the unconscious is often considered Involutionary, while the conscious is considered Evolutionary. Yet, to evolve we must become involved, so the two movements interact, exchange, and affect one another ceaselessly. This is shown in the interaction and mutual entwining of the serpents upon the Caduceus of Mercury.

3: **Element of Water**. A conscious intention must be *involved* to move the cycles of the Wheel to a higher octave, a change of speed, to *evolve*. This conscious intention must be combined with training knowledge and practice, as with any and all skills. Contrary to popular New Age dogma merely "intending" something to change is seldom sufficient. *We must also define and create the conditions whereby changes may manifest. Paradoxically this is not achieved by the will, as might be assumed, but by allowing the hidden seed of change, already present in all things, to germinate, grow, and manifest within defined* *parameters. The parameters offered are those of the Sphere of Art.*

4: **Element of Fire**. From a catalyzing substance we progress to the next level with an energizing force, the Earth Light, the telluric fire, rising from the heart of the planet, within the Sphere. This is met from above by the stellar fire. The *fusion* of these twin fires is essential to our evolutionary acceleration.

5: **Element of Air**. Here we come to Air as Spirit…the higher octave of the Elemental Cycle. This is the spiritual presence that emanates within a sealed and balanced Sphere of Art to evolve our chosen metals, minerals, elements, substances, and ultimately the mysterious collective of all of them, that we call ourselves.

Thus we can work through the ten Emanations (Spheres of the Tree) and their related manifestations, as described in *Aesch Mezareph*. These forms of emanation are the substances listed previously, as frequently defined in the septenary planetary traditions of Qabalah and Alchemy, activated through conscious work with the Tree of Life.

We are not, however, conducting physical experiments *upon* substances from outside (the classic method of material science that is often incorrectly applied to Alchemy), but conducting spiritual transformations from *within*. Not within the psyche, but within the vessel of the Sphere of Art, wherein the psyche is made still and void, like the first *Tohu* referred to in *Aesch Mezareph*, referring in turn to the famous creation verses of Genesis, all deriving from a pre-Christian, pre-Judaic mythic wisdom tradition. This same concept of Something coming from Nothing, of Cosmos from the Void, of Being from Un-being, is found in many spiritual traditions, and should not be thought of as solely originating in Biblical tradition.

We might take this a stage further, and suggest that we are, when empty and void, working *within* the catalyzing substances themselves, through their harmonic connection to each Emanation mirrored in miniature in the human body.

Practical Work (1)

The Dry Materials

A REMINDER: Before undertaking these practices, you should be familiar with the Tree of Life [11] and especially with the methods of the Sphere of Art [2]. The new practices will not work properly for you otherwise. Please consider carefully the following two preliminaries:

1 : You will experience the pleasant challenge of finding and assembling your metal and mineral samples, from the many sources available. Make this task of research, purchase and assembly a calm steady process, and do not rush. Ideally you should find small samples already provided in glass vials, though you may have to obtain some samples and vials separately.

2: There are two ways to undertake the practical work with the Dry and Wet materials. The first is with the physical substances as small metal and mineral samples. The second is with homeopathic potencies of these substances, which are easily found in most health-food stores or from on-line homeopathic suppliers. The homeopathic approach is described after the method of Elevation, which method is the same for both physical samples and homeopathic potencies of the traditional metals and minerals.

Beginning the Cycle

You are engaging in a conscious evolutionary movement that begins with the 10th Emanation or Kingdom, and moves from Earth and Moon, to Sun and Planets, to Stars. Working with the Dry materials as described, only a very small amount is needed. Ideally it should be powdered or in fine grains. Ten small identical air-tight and labeled vials are necessary for the work, enabling the substances to be moved and placed easily, or be exposed to light or kept in darkness as required.

NOTE: Mercury, the 8th metallic sample substance, is poisonous and must be handled carefully, and should always be kept in its vial. It appears to be a liquid, even when in its manifest or "solid" form. The old alchemists sometimes called it metallic mercury, as distinct from philosophic or qualitative Mercury, the Dry Water...combining both the Dry and Wet qualities. (Homeopathic Mercury is non-toxic).

Our example that follows, uses (10) carbon, as pure charcoal or sulfurous lava as the model for all ten substances. The ten substances must each be steadily worked through the ten stages of reverse emanation or exaltation, rising on the Tree of Life, within the Sphere of Art. This method requires that you work through all ten in each stage, before progressing to the next stage with all ten. This can be done with the physical substances, as described shortly, or with the homeopathic potencies of the same substances, as described at the close of the chapter.

Thus, to begin the cycle, substance 10, charcoal carbon, would be worked up the Tree from Emanation or Sphere 10 to Emanation 1.

Next 9, Silver, likewise, from 10 to 1. Then 8, Mercury, and so on, until all 10 substances have been individually elevated from the 10th Emanation to the 1st within the Sphere of Art. This simple process is easy to follow, and can be completed in a planned cycle, taking approximately 15 minutes per substance.

One of the "secrets" of *Aesch Mezareph* and similar methods is that we work from the Kingdom to the Crown, not the Crown to the Kingdom as described in the cosmic process from origination to creation, formation, and expression. We are *returning* thereby. Our return is enabled by the rising Earth Light, and received by the descending stellar forces; to us it seems that they fuse and merge with one another in the Sphere of Art around and within the substance or metal.

10: Begin with powdered charcoal carbon or lava (then the remaining nine substances in order 9-1).

10.1: Initially hold the substance in its vial, and meditate upon it. Make yourself Still, using the Stillness Chant **IAO** (described in Volume One), and discover the difference in feeling between carbon and lava: one is the organic basis for life on Earth; the other is the result of telluric fire, without which there is no life on Earth. Initially work with carbon for your first cycle, and then with lava for a second cycle, allowing time to rest after you have completed the first. The carbon cycle and the lava cycle will produce different results, and should not be mingled.

There are, therefore, two complete cycles, carbon and lava (closely associated with sulfur). You will have a total of twenty-two small vials when you have completed both cycles The numbers 10 and 22 are significant as the Ten Emanations and Twenty-Two Paths generating the Tree of Life. You may try various touch-sense communions with the substance, but do not ingest it, or try to absorb it through your skin. Usually the powdered material in a glass vial is the best way to attune to the subtle forces in their manifest or Kingdom octave.

10.2: Involves working through all ten Emanations with each substance in turn. Open the Sphere of Art, empty and seal the Sphere, and place the vial on a small stand or altar in the center. No other objects should be present on the altar. Be aware of the Sensitive Points below and above, and the twin fires or lights that merge in the substance. Make yourself very still using **IAO** as described in Volume One.

NOTE: Do not seek to "charge" or energize the substance through invocation. Allow the charge to occur through the twin fires that are *already present*, and are focused by the Sphere of Art. Let your awareness rest upon the material lightly, and be Still. Sense see and feel the twin fires, the Red and White Dragons, the Evolutionary and Involutionary tides at work, fusing together harmoniously around and through the material. Let it be itself through all worlds, all possibilities, and all states of being.

This central location and charging of the material in the Sphere must be done for each substance, in the order of reverse emanation, from 10-1, before you progress to the next stage. See Table One and the Lunar Cycle chart.

Do not jump ahead, or the cumulative effect of the work will not occur, and you will have to begin again. This is why old alchemical texts often describe how slow some processes are, how laborious, whereby patience is an essential requisite.

While this is indeed a spiritual allegory about working within and upon one's map (rather than the actual territory), it is also a true description; all transformation requires discipline and patience. Work through all ten, from Kingdom to Crown. This should be done at the rate of one substance per day, without fail. Taking a day off at any point during the cycle will break the cumulative effect, so plan ahead! If you are forced by circumstance to break, you must begin again. A complete cycle, starting with charcoal carbon, takes 11 days. The lava cycle would take a further 11 days and requires a new set of substances, either physical samples or homeopathic potencies.

Remember that charcoal or carbon is the prime substance for our kind of organic life, transformed by surface fire. Lava or volcanic ash is the core material of the planet transformed by telluric fire. The two cycles will elevate the metals, and yourself, in different ways.

The transformative processes cannot be rushed, skipped, or subverted. There is Qabalistic significance in the two eleven- day cycles. A single cycle equates to the Ten Emanations of the Tree of Life, plus the seed of Beginning for a new cycle. Two cycles give twenty two completed and elevated substances, the Paths of the Tree of Life.

NOTE: Do not invoke or meditate upon deities or images for the Emanations, for if you do so the entire process will fail. Our Sphere of Art/*Aesch Mezareph* method is not one of magical evocation or invocation [2].

Whichever substance you are working with embodies within itself the power of its Planet; the Planet expresses the higher spiritual octave of its originating Emanation. The substance, therefore, becomes *accelerated* through the subtle forces of the Sphere of Art.

Our task is to be still and enable this acceleration by allowing it to be, not to force it or enhance it, not to will it, not even to encase it in terms of imagery. As many contemporary practices involve visualization, and as sight is so over-emphasized in our culture, letting go of images can be surprisingly difficult. As always, the key is found in the Stillness meditation, stilling and letting go of Time, Space, and Events.

The Sphere of Art is primarily empty, and only by being empty of the Sub-Lunar forces can it fill, of its own accord, with the focused telluric and stellar forces. We must also remember to be empty and void within ourselves, as the historic text reminds us, like the first *Tohu*.

NOTE: the time required in each day may vary according to the chosen substance, some taking longer than others. Trust your intuitions and subtle senses within the Sphere; if you intuit that the process is complete for any one substance, be still, and ready to remove it from the altar. Typically you might allow up to 15 minutes maximum for each material, so with the opening, sealing, closing and releasing of the Sphere, the entire process, for one substance only, will probably last from 20 up to 30 minutes maximum. More may be excessive or unnecessary, but each individual will find his or her own pace.

10.3: Sit or stand in the center, holding the substance. Be aware of the Sensitive Points below and above. Feel the Earth Light and Stellar Fire come together in your body, circulating through both you and the substance. Come into deep communion with whatever share of that substance you have *within your body.*

Do not ingest the material, but instead feel for its counterpart within you, and begin to relate consciously to both the inner and outer material. Let the outer, charged with the twin fires and twin movements, catalyze the inner.

This third stage (10.3), with yourself in the center, should be undertaken with all ten materials. Working at the rate of one per day, through ten days of dedicated work. There is one more day to go.

10.4: Place all ten vials in the center, on the small stand or altar. Align them in a circle from 1-10, so that 10 (carbon or lava) is next to 1 (crystal or sulfur). As an alternative second process, after working with the Circle 1-10, you may also align them in a Tree of Life pattern, as shown in Figure Twelve, (The Pattern of the Vials). Remember, only small amounts of each substance should be used, and in equal amounts, a few grams or parts of each.

10.5: In a sealed Sphere of Art, go into Stillness. Let the New Sun fuse Above and Below in the center, around the constellation circle of all ten materials.

10.6: Create and extend your cord of connection to the center, coming from the Solar center of your body, likewise to the Sensitive Point above from the back of your neck, and the Sensitive Point below from the soles of your feet, as in Figure Thirteen. Remain Still in this communion for at least five minutes, no less [13]. *Withdraw gently from the communion, draw in the astral cord, and release the Sphere.*

Stages 10.4-6 will take one session only, one day. Thus we have a cycle of 11 days of dedicated work, initially with the carbon cycle. At a later date you would repeat the entire process, beginning with sulfurous lava, and nine new vials of the other substances. Your total will be two cycles, 22 days, with rest time between each cycle.

A Period of Rest

After each day cycle, take a break. You will often read or hear that ritual cycles should be synchronized with the Moon. This is especially important if you are engaged in Sub-Lunar realm practices. A typical synchronization for our reverse emanation would be to begin ten or eleven days before the full Moon, and if you undertake the entire double cycle (11 x2) it will end eleven days after full Moon. You may prefer to undertake the first cycle in one lunar month, and the second in the next month, working up to full Moon each time. *Whichever method you choose, be sure to take at least three days of rest after completion. The rest period may include keeping notes or a diary of impressions if you wish, but no other sacromagical or spiritual practices of any kind.*

This rest phase is essential for integration of the subtle forces. Do not take any mineral supplements or homeopathic remedies during the entire cycle, as your body must be clear of any modifying influences that might relate to the work in hand. During the cycle of work and the rest phase avoid any medications unless they are essential to support your life! Do not take any stimulants or alcohol! Eat lightly, try to sleep early and rise early.

A Lunar cycle is recommended, therefore, bearing in mind that our Sphere of Art practices do not include the forces of the Sub-Lunar realm, by the very nature of the art itself. A dedicated worker might wish to compare a cycle that is synchronized to the Moon, with a cycle that is started by picking a random date, perhaps by drawing lots.

Whatever way it is synchronized, an 11 day cycle, followed by a rest period is the pattern for working with both the Dry and Wet way. After the rest period at the end of the complete 22 part double cycle, you can return to your usual spiritual practices. Do not overdo the *Aesch Mezareph* practice, however, as this will be counter-productive.

You may combine the Dry and Wet Way in one 22 day cycle as shown in the preceding calendar chart. You should always do the Dry Way practice first as described, and after a rest period move on to the Wet Way practice that is described next. *Do not skip to the Wet Way cycle until you have completed the Dry Way cycle described above, as this will not work effectively for you.*

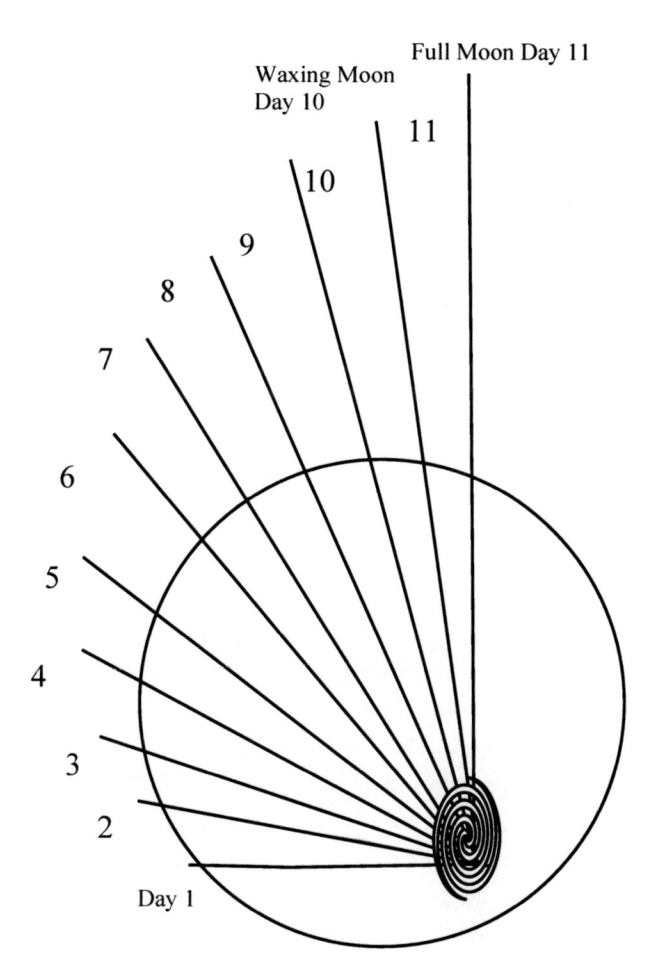

The Basic Cycle of Ten Days, plus the Collective Day.

Day 1:	Sphere 10	Kingdom	Earth
Day 2:	Sphere 9	Foundation	Moon
Day 3:	Sphere 8	Glory	Mercury
Day 4:	Sphere 7	Victory	Venus
Day 5:	Sphere 6	Beauty	Sun
Day 6:	Sphere 5	Severity	Mars
Day 7:	Sphere 4	Mercy	Jupiter
Day 8:	Sphere 3	Understanding	Saturn
Day 9:	Sphere 2	Wisdom	Neptune/Zodiac
Day 10:	Sphere 1	Crown	Uranus/Stars

85

Practical Work (2) The Wet Materials

The wet materials consist of energetic preparations of the ten primary substances, that you will enable, in small vials of pure water. These preparations are made from the Dry substances through energetic induction, on the altar, in the activated Sphere of Art. In this method water is potentized on the altar, by energetic induction from the materials that you have *already elevated* in the Dry substance stage, working with the Tree of Life as described above. The same process, with some minor practical adjustments, applies if you are using homeopathic potencies of the substances, and this is described at the end of the chapter.

Potentization in spring water is also the method use for preparing flower essences, which are homeopathic or energetic remedies from flowers, and for many other essences that are increasingly popular. In our method we usually do not immerse the ten subtly charged physical substances in the water. Typically the sample substance is kept next to the bowl of water, touching the side of the bowl. That is all that is necessary.

NOTE: At this stage we are working only with the ten primary materials as relating to the Spheres of the Tree of Life and their associated substances. If you truly wish this method to work, do not experiment outside its simple boundaries. Do not, for example, buy or prepare mixed essences that contain multiple substances for your work. Stay with the cycles as described.

One of the classic temptations in redemptive and transformative spiritual Alchemy, and indeed in all spiritual endeavors, is to try many possibilities once a method is understood. Resist this and calmly work within your Sphere of Art to evolve consciously the metals within you, within themselves, and at-one within the Sphere. This stage by stage acceleration process steadily dissolves the conditioned illusory map and enables you to return to the territory itself. If you try too much, too fast, too soon, you will undoubtedly fail, as with all skills, arts, and sciences. In Chapter Seven, analyzing the source text, we will find a similar caution couched in allegory, relating to *Gehazi* the

The Two Month Lunar Cycle.

The months of December to February are shown as examples.

	New Moon Cycle	Day	Moon	Full Moon Cycle	
		30-Dec		carbon	1
		31-Dec		silver	
		1-Jan	☽	mercury	
		2-Jan		copper	
		3-Jan		gold	
		4-Jan		iron	
		5-Jan		tin	
		6-Jan		lead	
		7-Jan		salt	
		8-Jan	○	sulphur	
		9-Jan	○	all	
		10-Jan	○	rest	
1	carbon	11-Jan		rest	
	silver	12-Jan		rest	
	mercury	13-Jan		lava	2
	copper	14-Jan		silver	
	gold	15-Jan	☾	mercury	
	iron	16-Jan		copper	
	tin	17-Jan		gold	
	lead	18-Jan		iron	
	salt	19-Jan		tin	
	sulphur	20-Jan		lead	
	all	21-Jan		salt	
	rest	22-Jan	●	sulphur	
	rest	23-Jan	●	all	
	rest	24-Jan	●	rest	
2	lava	25-Jan		rest	
	silver	26-Jan		rest	
	mercury	27-Jan			
	copper	28-Jan			
	gold	29-Jan			
	iron	30-Jan			
	tin	31-Jan	☽		
	lead	1-Feb			
	salt	2-Feb			
	sulphur	3-Feb			
	all	4-Feb			
	rest	5-Feb			
	rest	6-Feb	○		
	rest	7-Feb	○		
		8-Feb	○		

New Moon Cycle pivots around a period of rest at the height of the New Moon for the first set of metals/minerals.

Full Moon Cycle pivots around working the All at the height of the Full Moon for the first set of metals/minerals.

servant of the prophet Elisha. This servant's name means "valley of avarice".

There are two ways of working with the wet materials: potentizing them individually in the center of the Sphere, and potentizing them further, collectively, (all ten at once) in the center of the Sphere. These further potentizings require fresh spring water or any clean water that you trust...distilled water could be used if necessary. Pure spring water is best.

The Single Method

In the single method the vial and a small bowl of spring water are placed in the center. Do not put the substance directly into the water. Within your sealed Sphere of Art, let the twin fires work on the water and the material together. Afterwards, use the water (only) as the matrix to prepare an essence as described in Appendix One.

NOTE: Traditionally work of this sort was undertaken after consulting an ephemeris or making observations of the planetary relationships. If, for example, there was a difficult aspect to the chosen planet and its related metal you might not work with it until that aspect had improved.

Another traditional method was to work with the Chaldean Planetary Hours, and this can be helpful for Sphere of Art work, though it is not essential. The late A.R. Heaver was a sidereal astrologer, but he also worked with the Chaldean Planetary Hours, according to notes in my possession.

In this method the single substance is worked with during its appropriate Planetary Hour. Accurate Planetary Hours depend upon your location, and fortunately you can find Planetary Hour calculators, defined by location, on several astrological websites. For example: you are working with silver, the Foundation or 9th Emanation, the Moon. Find the Planetary Hours for the Moon in your cycle, and work with one of them. You would repeat this for all ten materials as described in our list above, during the appropriate hours for each Planet. The Planetary Hours may be attuned to during the day or at night, so this allows some flexibility in planning your schedule.

The Collective Method

The collective method uses a small bowl of spring water in the center, with the ten previously charged substance vials constellated around it in sequence from 1-10, so 10 is next to 1, or as shown in Figure Twelve (The Pattern of the Vials). Planetary Hours for this Collective Method follow the Middle Pillar of the Tree of Life, so you would plan ahead according to the cycle of the planetary hours in any one day as appropriate for your location.

1st Hour, earliest threshold of dawn

2nd Hour, Sun

3rd Hour, Moon

4th Hour, Earth (this last of the Four Hours is your choice of time to conclude the work).

Planetary Hours relate to the Wanderers or Seven Planets, so there is no "hour" for the Crown/Uranus, or for Wisdom/Neptune. They could be embodied in their lower manifest octaves, the Crown-Uranus resonating through Beauty and the Sun, and Wisdom-Neptune, resonating through Mercy- Jupiter, but in our method the first moment of dawn stands for the Crown, Uranus, and Spirit, and your human choice of timing for the last hour stands for the Kingdom of Earth and Manifestation.

As before, the result will be a matrix for an essence, in this case a tenfold constellated Tree of Life essence, with the Planetary Hours attuning the Middle Pillar from Stars to Sun to Moon to Earth.

Conclusion: The Dry Way, the Wet Way, the Elevation

There are three stages to the elevation or exaltation of the substances or *materia*.

1: **The Dry Way**. The chosen substances, either physical samples or homeopathic potencies thereof, are progressively exalted from the Kingdom to the Crown. The Rising Earth Light and Descending Starlight, embodied by the Red and White Dragons, transform the material during its progressive elevation from Earth to the Stars. In conclusion you will have ten small vials of highly charged samples of Carbon, Silver, Mercury, Copper, Gold, Iron, Tin, Lead, Salt, and Sulphur/Crystal. If you repeat the cycle with sulfurous lava as your Kingdom material, you will have twenty small vials, a carbon set and a lava set. A further collective Elevation for each gives twenty-two vials.

2: **The Wet Way**. The charged tenfold materials (from either the carbon cycle or the lava cycle, but not both at once) are elevated again, *one at a time*, while touching a small bowl of pure water. The water receives its first potentization from the charged substances. Thus you will conclude with ten charged samples of water, one from each new bowl of water for each Emanation or Planet. A portion of each of the ten waters should be carefully bottled and labeled. They form the matrices for further potentization as essences, according to Appendix One. Any excess should be offered to the land where you live, ideally pouring it during its appropriate Planetary Hour. If you are using homeopathic potencies of the substances, this method requires a slight variation, as described at the end of the chapter.

3: **Further Elevations**. The potentized waters can be further diluted and elevated. The more dilutions and elevations through the Emanations, the more powerful each essence becomes. You may do the same for the tenfold constellation of materials, as described above. In conclusion you will have ten matrix bottles (that will last for many years) and ten dilution bottles for practical use, plus another matrix and dilution for the tenfold constellated essence.

The Dry Way has a unique resonance for the Earth and Moon Foundational realms, for this is where the materials have their manifest life. This is the First Elevation. Do not proceed further until you have completed it successfully. If you break this cycle, for any reason, you must return to the beginning and start afresh.

The first Wet Way cycle has a unique resonance for the Sun and Planetary realms, for this is where the subtle forces permeate toward manifestation in the Foundational realm. This is the

Second Elevation, and must be fully completed before moving on the next stage.

A second Wet Way cycle is possible (i.e. a third cycle) has a uniquely stellar resonance. This is the Third Elevation, and is the last phase of the work.

Working with the Results

When this process is described, people often say "very well, I understand it. But what am I supposed to do with all these little vials of metals and liquid? The answer is "You will have already done it", the Elevation is everything. Nevertheless, we can offer some suggestion for practical use of the vials.

Your collection of vials can be placed together one or more small boxes . You can meditate with each sample in turn, or by combining them. While single samples embody the Emanations through the metal or substance, combinations will embody Paths and Triads of the Tree of Life. Thus gold and copper will embody the Path associated with The Lovers, Sun and Venus, Beauty and Victory. The complete list of metals and tarot images is shown in Appendix Five [36].

Using Homeopathic Potencies of the Materials

You may also elevate the materials through equivalent samples of potentized homeopathic preparations. Homeopathy has many historical and conceptual relationships to Alchemy. The homeopathic principle involves exponentially high dilutions of a substance creating resonances that can act in a curative manner in the human body. Many of the core homeopathic remedies are based upon the traditional attributes of the Seven Planets, the minerals, and their transformations through heat, solution, and amalgamation. albeit with thousands of other remedies in use today.

A list of homeopathic equivalents is given at the end of this section. Ideally "6x" potencies should be used, and these can be obtained from homeopathic pharmacies on-line. In health stores most remedies are found in the "30c" potency, and this can also be used. The 6x potency is closer to the physical substance in nature, while the higher potencies are further from it due to exponential dilutions.

The Dry Way: In this alternative method, small homeopathic pills or tablets are used instead of the ten material substances . Use four pills only for each . The pills should be dispensed from their supply container directly into your ten glass vials without touching them by hand. Follow all the standard homeopathic cautions for keeping remedies untainted.

The Wet Way: Using your previously Elevated set of homeopathic equivalents, dissolve one pill (only) from each substance in pure water. Simply fill each glass vial with a pre-prepared blend of 1/3 alcohol (as a preservative, use a good quality vodka or, ideally, a bio-dynamic brandy) and 2/3 pure water, mixed well together. Leave a small space for adding the single pill. In the Collective method, dissolve all ten samples (one pill of each substance) in a sealed container of pre-mixed alcohol and pure water. Place this in the center of the Sphere, as in our standard method. NOTE: the pills may dissolve slowly, but their subtle resonance will rapidly permeate the water. Never touch the pills by hand: you may choose to use a pair of clean tweezers dedicated for the purpose.

List of equivalent remedies at 6x or 30c: use the same potency throughout, and do not mix 6x and 30c potencies:

1 Sulphur: Sulphur

2 Salt: Natrum Muriaticum (Nat. Mur.)

3 Lead: Plumbum Metallicam (Plumbum)

4 Tin: Stannum Metallicum

5 Iron: Ferrum Metallicum

6 Gold: Aurum Metallicum (Aurum)

7 Copper: Cuprum Metallicum

8 Mercury: Mercurius Vivus (Merc. Viv.)

9 Silver: Argentum Metallicum (Argent. Met.)

10: Carbon: Carbo Vegetabilis (Carbo Veg)

(10: Lava: Hekla Lava, an established remedy, or Etna Lava, a more recently potentized remedy)

Several remedies have variant combinations, such as Ferrum Phos., Argent. Nit.,Nat. Sulph, and so on. Use only the metallic and salt remedies listed above, which still hold the subtle resonance of the original metals and minerals.

In Chapter Four we will explore a potent method of further enhancing the entire process of transforming the metals and elements within ourselves and within Nature. This is the Mystery of the Four Holy Fires.

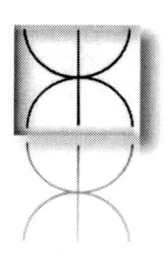

CHAPTER FOUR

The Four Holy Fires

The Four Holy Fires can be instituted as a daily practice; this form improves exponentially at first, then after rapid early results, stabilizes and continues to develop steadily and clarify over time. It can take as little as five minutes, or can be extended for a longer period. Once a day would be sufficient, but ideally it can be done at dawn and dusk as a general practice. Another significant time for the Four Holy Fires is true midnight...the middle of the night hours, found by calculation, between sunset and sunrise. For this practice you should sleep before your work with the Four Holy Fires, set a gentle alarm for the calculated mid-night, then go to sleep again after you have completed your five to ten minutes of practice.

Working with the Four Holy Fires greatly benefits the Elevation of the Metals described in Chapter Three. It should, however, be practiced first as a form in its own right, before combining it with the elevation of substances or metals. Once you are practiced in the Four Holy Fires, they can be combined with the form for elevating each substance as follows:

1: Elevate the chosen substance as described. For example, take Silver and Moon in the reverse emanation pattern, from the Kingdom to the Crown, a cycle of ten workings. Each time you pause to commune with the metal within an Emanation (i.e. Silver in any one of the Emanations as it is ascending) work through the Four Holy Fires within your body. Always remember to return to Stillness.

2: After a full experience of (1) above, with all ten substances through the Ten Emanations, work with the Four Holy Fires for the overall Tree of Life and the metals or substances. This is shown in Figure Fourteen (The Four Holy Fires).

The Four Holy Fires is an advanced method that follows from The Rising Light exercise found in *Earth Light* and *Power Within the Land* [4]. While you can work immediately with the Four Holy

Fires from the instructions given here, practicing the Rising Light form first is highly recommended as a foundation.

Moving the Four Holy Fires within the Elemental Body

Earth: Feet and Legs
Water: Loins and Genitals
Fire: Lungs and Heart
Air: Head, Around and Above Head.

The Four Roots or Elements do not exist in abstract, but within one another. Thus Fire is whatever is primarily fiery in nature, and may have relative proportions of Earth, Water, and Air, within it. This interactive or interleaved relationship is self-iterating, resting upon the same mathematical principles as the popular fractal images shown visually on a computer screen. The principles of self-iteration were well-known in metaphysics, long before number-crunching machines revealed the visual beauty of the fractal image. Indeed, the Tree of Life is one such self-iteration, while the cycle of the Elements, rooted within one-another, expresses the same reality.

The Four Holy Fires are relative states or conditions of subtle Fire moving through the body. They have many expressions as bio-electrical and subtle energies, but in sacromagical practice we are concerned with their *movement* more than with the scientific or other definitions that vary from century to century and culture to culture.

Rising from the UnderWorld

The fiery energy begins within the planet, for it is the telluric fire or Earth Light, supporting all life on Earth. It does not begin in the human body, though the body is energized and transformed by it. As Earth Light rises through us, we consciously attune to the Elements in their native zones of the body, Earth for feet and legs, Water for genitals and pelvis, Fire for heart and lungs, and Air for mouth, head, and above the head, as in Figure Fourteen (The Four Holy Fires). Thus this form is not about working with "chakras" or stimulating one's own personal internal forces through focusing upon them. Such practices, though widespread and popular, are essentially self-indulgent and can progressively promote solipsistic isolation and self-focus more readily than communion and interaction.

Instead of focusing upon ourselves, we make ourselves Still, and the ever-present all-pervading Earth Light is invited to permeate the body according to the Four Zones, rising steadily through each zone. In response our inner energies willingly and spontaneously change. Note that the changes within us come through interaction with a planetary spiritual power, not through willpower, personal sexuality, or other ego-enhancing methods. As always in *Aesch Mezareph* practices, we must be still, void, clear, and empty. Only then will we experience true spiritual transformation.

We can work with Fire of Earth, Fire of Water, Fire of Fire, and Fire of Air in an ascending sequence as follows:

1: Be Still, stilling Time Space and Movement. Chant **OAI**. Align to, and affirm, the Seven Directions, as in Figure

2: Let your awareness rest upon the soles of your feet, which must be touching the earth or the floor that is in contact with the earth.

3: Follow that contact downwards into planet Earth, envisioning two lines or luminous cords, one from each foot. They twine together as they descend, becoming a single cord reaching deep into the core of the Earth. Be still, and feel this cord extend far beneath you. It is always present, but we are seldom conscious of it. In practice we tend to lose sight of the cord as it merges with the Earth Light below, but we can sense it or feel it nevertheless.

4: Sense see and feel the Earth Light respond and begin to ascend the cord, radiating upwards into your feet. Do not invoke, will, or concentrate upon the Earth Light. Instead, feel that the natural rising movement (actually a complex physical and metaphysical radiation that permeates everything unceasingly), responds to your lightest touch of awareness. The action is more like an allowing, a conversation, and a welcome recognition. As described in Chapter Two, the spiritual forces are naturally scaled-down by mediating entities and filters, so that we can work safely with them...no amount of will-power or invocation will change this. The scaled-down forces, however, are far greater than our normal interactions, and providing they are balanced through the methods described, will have powerful transformative energizing effects within us.

Around your feet legs and thighs, sense, see, and feel, a mobile swirling sphere of light: this is Fire of Earth. Pause and feel the subtle forces, meditate upon the nature of Fire of Earth, and feel how it works within you.

Initially spend a longer time upon each of the Fires, until you are familiar with them. Then you may work with the rising sequence more rapidly.

5: Allow this subtle Fire to rise steadily into the hips and genitals. Sense, see, and feel a second mobile sphere of light, somewhat merged with the first, and evolving out of it. This is Fire of Water. Its intensity increases. Pause and feel the subtle forces, meditate upon the nature of Fire of Water, and feel how it works within you.

6: Allow the subtle Fire to rise again steadily into the chest, lungs and heart. The third mobile sphere of light, merged somewhat with the second, and evolving out of the previous two fires, is Fire of Fire. It is the most intense thus far. Pause and feel the subtle forces, meditate upon the nature of Fire of Fire, and feel how it works within you.

7: Allow the subtle Fire to rise more rapidly to the Head and around your head. It evolves and accelerates from the previous three fires. This is Fire of Air. Its intensity is high and vibrant. Pause and feel the subtle forces, meditate upon the nature of Fire of Air, and feel how it works within and around you.

8: Affirm the Sacred Directions. Before you (East), behind you (West), right of you (South) left of you (North), above your head, beneath your feet, and the source of all-Being, within. Be still and feel how the Four Holy Fires interact, merge, and flow within your body.

8a: Discover how they interact with their counterparts in the planetary directions, Air in the East, Fire in the South, Water in the West, and Earth in the North. (This can be expanded into a separate form for regular practice).

9: Gently let the Fires descend from Air to Fire, Fire to Water, Water to Earth, down through the four zones of your body, Head, Heart, Genitals, and Feet. Feel their intensity diminish, but not fade entirely.

10: Be aware again of your feet upon the Earth, and of your body in relationship to the space around you, returning to your outer awareness.

The Combustion Cycle

The ascent of the Four Holy Fires can be compared, in a broad sense, to the cycle of combustion. This is not intended as a "scientific" comparison, but as a conceptual model of the transformation of energy inherent in the traditional idea of the Four Roots or Elements, beginning with earthy substance and transforming through increasing heat into incandescent airs, gases, or radiations.

1: Fire of Earth, whereby a substance is heated until its temperature rises. Or its potential internal fire may open and increase. The Earth that has been relatively cold and firm becomes warm and malleable as its Water is released. In the human body this concept begins with a meditation on the feet and legs, but passes through the entire substance of bones, fluids, flesh, and subtle forces. Note that the initiating energy begins *outside* the body, in the planetary body beneath the feet. The catalyzing or initiating fire, the Earth Light, triggers a response in the subtle forces *within*, which will radiate through the entire body.

2: Fire of Water, whereby increasing heat causes evaporation, increased release of moisture, humidity, fluid warmth. At its peak, Fire of Water can come to the boil. The connection to sexual arousal and generation and fertility is obvious and well-known, but this Fire of Water also modulates many aspects of the health and the internal organs of assimilation and elimination.

3: Fire of Fire, whereby increasing heat, ascending temperature, causes the substance to catch alight. Flame, radiant light and heat, incandescence begins. The body zone here is that of the heart working together with the lungs.

4: Fire of Air, at which stage gases are given off as the substance is transformed by fire. The peak temperature and incandescence possible, the most subtle yet potent energy is generated and released. The Element of Air moves beyond gases toward a higher octave of incandescence, emitting light as its earthy form is moved to the highest rate. Thus it radiates around the throat, and above and around the head. (This is the nimbus or halo that is often shown in iconography).

Note that each Element can be cold, warm, hot, or radiant, corresponding to Earth, Water, Fire, and Air. Thus cold water would be earthy, warm water would be watery, hot water fiery, and radiant water (steam and beyond) would be airy. This simple pattern can be meditated upon for each Element, generating many insights and subtle changes of energy and consciousness. None of these conditions are absolutes, and are intended to show the conceptual relativity of the Elements rather than act as scientific "definitions". The astrological model of the Triplicities (See Figure Ten) is an ancient expression of the same concept of relative interaction, and should be studied carefully as the traditional background to working with the Four Holy Fires.

After the relative combustion has peaked, there is a descending cycle from Head to Feet that can be likened to a steadily declining fire after its peak. The elements of the substances have changed due to the combustion cycle, yet they are not destroyed, only re-formed into new relationships and appearances. This simple sequence was one of the most important alchemical contemplations, often reinforced by repeated practical experiment. In our metaphysical work, we replicate the phoenix, for the energies are born anew from the ashes, when we begin each new cycle of the Four Holy Fires.

After exploring and experiencing the Four Holy Fires, we can begin to explore and work with the related *Affinities*. The Affinities are further sources for meditation and communion.

The Primary Affinities

The *Primary Affinities* correspond to the Middle Pillar of the Tree of Life as follows:

10: Carbon or Lava, Earth and Kingdom, Feet and legs, Fire of Earth. Archangel *Sandalphon* (feet of *Metatron*).

9: Silver, Moon and Foundation, Loins, pelvis, and genitals, Fire of Water. Archangel *Gabriel*, (androgynous genitals of *Metatron*).

6: Gold, Sun and Beauty, Heart and Lungs, Fire of Fire, Archangel *Michael* (Heart of *Metatron*).

1: Crystalline Sulphur or Quartz, Uranus and Crown, Head and mouth, Above Head, Fire of Air (Archangel *Metatron*).

There are four parts of the body in the *Primary Affinities*, Feet, Genitals, Heart, and Head, corresponding to the Middle Pillar of the Tree of Life, and the cosmic nesting of Earth, Moon, Sun, and Stars. Each of these four parts is central to the right and left parts of the *Secondary Affinities*.

The Secondary Affinities

The *Secondary Affinities* correspond to the Right and Left Hand Pillars:

<u>Right Hand Pillar</u> (when actively standing within the Tree of Life facing outwards with the Tree within or behind you, not when looking at a diagram or facing a representation of the Tree).

10: Carbon or Lava, Earth and Kingdom, Feet and legs, especially right leg. Fire of Earth. Archangel *Sandalphon* (feet of *Metatron*)

8: Quicksilver (mercury), Mercury and Scintillation, Glory, or Honor. Right hip and hand of organization and intelligence. Fire of Water, Archangel *Raphael*

5: Iron, Mars and Severity. Right arm. Fire of Fire, Archangel *Khamael*. Traditionally the sword arm or arm of just action.

3: Lead, Saturn, Understanding. Right shoulder. Fire of Air, Archangel *Tzaphkiel*.

NOTE: (3) and (8) may be interchangeable, pivoting around (5). This is a powerful Qabalistic exercise, related to the *Qabalah of the Three Suns* described in The Miracle Tree (book and CD) [11].

<u>Left Hand Pillar</u> (when standing within the Tree of Life)

10: Carbon or Lava, Earth and Kingdom, Feet and legs, especially left leg. Fire of Earth. Archangel *Sandalphon* (feet of *Metatron*).

7: Copper, Venus and Exaltation (Victory, Power) Left hip and hand of creativity and giving. Fire of Water, Archangel *Auriel*.

4: Tin, Jupiter and Mercy. Fire of Fire, Archangel *Tzadkiel*. Left arm. Traditionally the Staff or Rod Arm, but can also hold the Cup. The arm of generous action.

2: Salt, Neptune or Zodiac, Wisdom. Left shoulder. Fire of Air, Archangel *Ratziel*.

NOTE: (2) and (7) may be interchangeable, pivoting around (4). This is a powerful Qabalistic exercise, related to the *Qabalah of the Three Suns* described in The Miracle Tree (book and CD) [11].

The Secondary Affinities: there are nine combined-parts of the body in the *Secondary Affinities*.

1-2: Feet and Legs. (right and left, two parts). Discover that they are One when standing still and at Peace in the Kingdom or Territory, but become Two in action, with Movement, Right and Left. Movement is active and horizontal in any Direction across the Kingdom or territory. Peace is poised, still, and vertical, at the center within the Kingdom or territory. Understanding of this interaction dissolves the map, but lack of Understanding rigidifies the map.

3-4: Hips, loins, genitals, and corresponding hands (right and left, two parts). Discover that they are Two in action, with Movement, but are One when united at Peace. The Movement is alternative Right and Left, working either with or against one another. The Peace is horizontal, but together at Rest, above the Kingdom territory. One hand crossed over the other, palms downwards. This is the way of Blessing and giving forth that enables us to read beneath the surface of the Map without eyes or restless mind.

5-6: Arms and chest (right and left, two parts). Discover that they are Two in action, with Movement, but are joined as one by the Union of the Hands blessing the territory. The action or Movement of the arms is Horizontal, alternative Right and Left, working either with or against one another. Peace is Vertical, from Above to Below (shoulders to arms united by joined hands). The arms may also lift the hands, so that they are Joined as One above the Head. This is the way of Harmony with the joined hands below and above making the Hexagram.

7-8: Shoulders and above (right and left, two parts). Discover that they are Two in action as the sources of primary motion for the arms and hands. All poise and Peace in the body begins with the shoulders, bringing arms and hands, legs and feet, into Stillness.

9: Head and above head. (one part) Discover that the Head and Above is One in both Movement and Stillness. Let the Head balance all parts through Peace, and not the parts imbalance the head through distracted movement.

Summary of Practices Utilizing Aesch Mezareph

This concludes the practical work, which can be summarized thus:

1 Practice the Sphere of Art as described in Volume One, and in the supporting audio CD.

2 Work with the cycles of elevation, transforming the substances metals and Elements as described in Chapter Three. Two cycles as described over a period of days.

3 After having completed at least two cycles of elevating the substances, preferably several double cycles (i.e. 2,4,6,8 etc.) move on to working with The Four Holy Fires.

4 Practice the Four Holy Fires until you are familiar with them. Combine the Fires with the cycles of elevation, for at least two cycles or preferably multiples of two. You may use the materials

that you have previously elevated, and/or you may use new materials.

5 Discover the Affinities, and work with them separately until you have experienced them all and have become familiar with the patterns and the subtle forces that are generated.

6: Combine the Affinities with the Four Holy Fires and the elevation cycle, for at least two cycles or multiples of two. As before, you may use the materials that you have previously elevated, and/or new materials.

NOTE: Do not "drop" any part of any cycle or form. If you do so, you should begin again at stage one. A helpful method is to keep a simple work-chart. Discover how long a full cycle can take you, and how long a form, such as the Four Holy Fires or one of the Affinities sequences, can take you. From this draw-up a work-chart and schedule, and you will be able to calculate the timing for a full cycle within the Lunar phases and Planetary Hours. While this may seem daunting to read initially on the printed page, it is a simple process in practice

Once you have practiced the various modules or components, the full cycles start to flow naturally, and are easily remembered and recovered. Always work from memory, and not by turning pages. Text is helpful at first, but can never be a substitute for living memory. Memory-storage machines such as laptops or smart-phones must not be used or be present anywhere within the Sphere of Art, or in the room where you are working. Turn off all electrical appliances, and ideally isolate the physical space by turning off the power supply itself. This is usually recommended in subtle work because the quartz pulsing and other frequencies used in such technology may interfere with the subtle forces. With Sphere of Art work, however, there is always the possibility that hi-tech items, always notoriously neurotic and unreliable in behavior, will be fried by the subtle forces. The same applies to talismans, amulets, and previously empowered magical objects: they will be wiped clean within the Sphere of Art, so if you have such things, you might wish keep them separate from your Sphere of Art work.

The Cord and the Sphere

One tool or implement that can be used within the Sphere of Art is the spirit cord. Traditionally this would be a red cord, though you might also choose to use white or black. Some people prefer a dedicated red cord for their Fire Temple and Sphere of Art work. Methods for empowering a cord are described in detail in *The Spirit Cord* [13].

In Chapter Five we will explore the implications for working with the Tree of Life within the Sphere of Art.

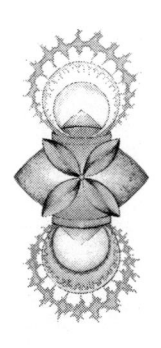

CHAPTER FIVE

The Tree of Life Within the Sphere of Art

One of the questions often asked, regarding Sphere of Art practice, is "how might we work with the Emanations of the Tree of Life within the Sphere of Art?" To answer this question, we can explore the interaction of metaphysics and methods within the Sphere of Art. By exploring this interaction first in words, then in practice, we can improve and accelerate our sacromagical work. In addition to elevation of the metals, there are other forms that may be experienced within the sealed Sphere. As always, upon this path, the more simple the form, the more powerful its effect. Some of the potential problems of excessive complexity are explored in this chapter, and some solutions offered toward simplicity.

Elucidation of the Sphere of Art

The Sphere of Art is an alchemical vessel of energy and consciousness, though it may not be found in a physical laboratory. The stages of practice in our previous chapters reveal a middle-ground between outer alchemical physical and inner withdrawn metaphysical work. Practitioners may also choose to work with practical Alchemy in the laboratory, but this is not required or necessary for the subtle transformations that are enabled by the practice of *Aesch Mezareph* within the Sphere of Art.

Practical laboratory work was regarded as essential for those of a certain elemental characteristic, or, to put it more simply, who needed a physical hands-on approach. Spiritual traditions worldwide, all have a physical component especially suited for those who find enlightenment through practical physical work. Ideally physical interaction should be combined with spiritual endeavor, and our methods for experiencing *Aesch Mezareph, Purifying Fire*, combine simple alchemical processes with the subtle forces within the Sphere of Art. In laboratory Alchemy there is a strong emphasis upon physical fire, while in the Sphere of Art the emphasis is upon spiritual fire. Upon either path of fire, repeated practice and dedication is required.

The Sphere of Art is a unique practice within itself, whereby the transcendent laboratory is built from the interaction between the body and certain well-defined spiritual forces that may be generated within the Sphere, or may enter it from metaphysical sources, often called the Inner Planes, but not implying a merely psychological ground. The Sphere of Art is built not within the mind, not inside the skull, but by shaping subtle forces around the practitioner who works undisturbed in a defined enclosed physical space. This is a mirroring of the process called "hewing out" in some poetic translations of Qabalistic sources, using an analogy to the human skills of carving or shaping with the hands, or with a tool or blade. In the *Sefer Yetzirah* [14] time, space, and spiritual movement (energy) are hewn by the prime Being, sculpted into the essential Seven Directions that enable manifestation. As with all poetic wisdom teachings, a few words contain a wealth of implication.

Teaching and Transmission

The relationship between the Tree of Life and the Sphere of Art is, in fact, often described in the wide spectrum of older magical, alchemical, and Qabalistic literature, though seldom understood, and rarely given a clear exposition. As with many esoteric methods, there are fragments available in plain view, but they are not often seen, and there is seldom any guidance on piecing the fragments together.

As always, an oral wisdom tradition is missing from the published texts, and the student is supposed to receive further teaching by direct transmission. Within the gradual evolution of esoteric initiatory and transformative traditions new methods of working appear, based upon the wisdom of the past. This is the model found in this book; the wisdom of the past is our foundation, upon which new techniques are built. Often the apparent boundary between "old" and "new" is soft, as we are working with consciousness rather than precisely dated records. Nevertheless the new forms and ways of working can be defined, in context of traditional sources, and presented as practical methods. Thus the new outer methods can be described initially in a book or essay, and can be substantially helped by an audio recording. The practice itself, as always, is the responsibility of the student.

The audio recording is an important modern development, because it occupies a place half-way between written teachings and oral elucidation. On the *Sphere of Art* and *Miracle Tree* CDs that support the earlier books in this series, the empowered visionary forms can be heard as they are *actively* practiced, within the Sphere of Art. In this way, some of the subtle effect is transmitted through the voice and music, reaching beyond a constructed recording of a recital or dramatic performance.

It should be emphasized that the Sphere of Art is *a* Qabalah, within the overall tradition of *The* Qabalah, and is essentially a Hermetic or Neo-Platonic Qabalah. By this we simply mean that it is a special development within the broad and deep Western stream of esoteric tradition, and derived Jewish mystical tradition alone. Please remember that in this book the Jewish traditions are spelled Kabbalah, while the Western or Hermetic traditions are spelled Qabalah. None of these distinctions are of great import, as the three main streams, Jewish, Muslim (Sufi), and Hermetic share many common origins in the ancient world. This threefold interaction of the traditional cultural Qabalah(s) is discussed further in *The Miracle Tree* [11].

Qabalistic traditions are received wisdom, "from mouth to ear" or whispered. While this refers to verbal instruction or elucidation given to initiates, it also refers to the whispers that are heard, but not with ears. Such whispers are the intimations that arise in deep spiritual communion, and these must be carefully compared to material in the received outer tradition. Appendix Two on *Inner Contacts* explores this process further.

I received the main form and practice of *The Sphere of Art* from my Inner Contacts, while working from a series of cryptic clues given by the late Alfred Ronald Heaver, though I did not understand them until some years after his death. Within the three main streams of Qabalistic tradition (Hebrew, Hermetic, Sufi) there are many individual Qabalahs or "whispered wisdom" traditions and methods. The Sphere of Art and its associated tradition of *Aesch Mezareph* as we practice it, is a Hermetic Qabalah, deriving from sources such as, but not limited to, Hebrew *Kabbalah* and the broader spectrum of Qabalah in general.

Sphere of Art Qabalah, therefore, is a special practice that derives in part from Pythagorean, Empedoclean, Platonic, and Neo-Platonic sources, in part due to the geometric patterns involved, and in part due to the wide streams of philosophy and metaphysics associated with such names. Many scholars have explored the interaction of philosophical and metaphysical traditions in the ancient world, but here we are concerned less with history than with living practice.

In the context of origins, we should always remember that the connections within the perennial spiritual traditions are more than a history or time-line of texts. While ancient sources are essential as training, and as proof, within a tradition, they are never linear in the sense of literary history. More simply, the core spiritual traditions are all based on a shared consciousness that arises when humans turn away from ephemeral worldly pursuits and fix attention on the Stars and on the spiritual origins of the cosmos.

Such insights as may come are shared through the centuries, not only in texts or teaching, but in repeated experience. The cultural or ethnic dress will vary substantially, especially between Eastern and Western (Northern) traditions, but the inner truths and transformations are at a deeper level and tend to support one another wherever they are found around the world.

The Sphere of Art as an initiatory path is supported, nourished, and maintained through the centuries by a hidden ongoing Western esoteric tradition within specific alchemical and practical sacromagical or theurgic lineages handed down by direct initiation. I received this initiation from both W G Gray (1913-1992) and A R Heaver (1900-1980) each of whom embodied different branches of the tradition.

This hidden tradition includes, but is not limited to, esoteric methods described in the alchemical text *Aesch Mezareph* and metaphysics as described in the major Qabalistic source text, *Sefer Yetzirah*. Varying scholarly opinions date this source text anywhere between the second century BCE and the second century CE, but whatever the exact date of writing that will never be known, it reports an established metaphysical tradition and practice. Like all such threshold texts, it was written out long after oral tradition and initiatory practice was well established, and consists of basic teachings and notes intended for further elucidation. *Sefer Yetzirah* is widely available in free editions on internet archives, or in published editions with commentaries that vary in quality. Probably the best modern edition and commentary, and undoubtedly the most thorough and complete in English, is that of Aryeh Kaplan [1].

The Physical Space: The Temple Not Built With Hands

The Sphere of Art is a microcosm of the "temple not built with hands" that is referred to in esoteric tradition and texts. As we are living within space and time, on planet Earth, we begin by honoring, embracing, and including, the spatial dimensions.

The physical space should ideally be a room or small building that is not used for anything else, as, with repeated use, it gradually and progressively intersects with metaphysical locations and spiritual energies. As a vessel, the energetic Sphere of Art, which is built within the physical space, becomes the true place of transformation, comparable to the alembic or alchemical spherical vessel containing the *materia* used in physical alchemical experiments. For energy to initiate transformation, it must be contained, force within form. This basic law can be moved through octaves, until the form is, in itself, no longer a manifest shell, but an octave of force, and the force generated within that octave is of a new kind, perceived and felt through a transformation of our consciousness. Modern physics has taught us afresh, through new models, that there is no firm matter, only relative states of energy. Such an understanding is not, as we are often led to believe "new", for has always been inherent to magical, theurgic, or alchemical practices, albeit presented in allegorical, gnomic, or mystical terminology. The understanding is perennial, only the models of expression change through the centuries. A classic and increasingly popular model is that of Sacred Geometry.

Sacred Geometry

With repeated practice a dedicated physical space will remain attuned for long periods of time. We can find evidence of this long term process not only in the geometric design of ancestral sacred sites (which has attracted so much frivolous attention in recent years that it has been overlaid with a crust of New Age dogma) but in our direct perception of subtle forces. What is popularly called "sacred geometry" should be combined with conscious intention growing understanding, and not simply copied from diagram to diagram without inner elucidation. It is often assumed in contemporary practice that to copy some geometric patterns, by planting stones or making a labyrinth, or burying crystals, into the land, will cause spiritual or energetic transformation without any effort by humans. This approach is materialistic, a mechanistic "quick-fix" illusion, identical to the notion that by speaking incomprehensible "Words of Power" aloud the self-styled magician can command supernatural forces. None of this nonsense will suffice for serious spiritual transformation.

We should combine the outer patterns of geometry with the inner patterns of geometry. Unless we have a deep meditative and energetic communion with the cosmic shapes as they manifest, they will be mere decoration, a matter of esthetics rather than a living shape mediating between dimensions of being. In some examples, so-called "sacred geometry" creates a markedly unhealthy influence upon the land, as it is installed without harmonious relationship and understanding, becoming an imposition rather than a conscious co-creation.

Threefold Interaction Within a Physical Space

Repeated practice rapidly discovers a threefold interaction or interleaving in the creation of the Sphere of Art.

1: The first zone of interaction is the chosen physical space. This seems at first to be only an outer shell, a set of boundaries, the manifest space defined by the Sub-Lunar realm of Nature, within which the subtle Sphere is generated. Later we will experience some remarkable effects of defining such a zone.

The Sphere can be generated outdoors, of course, but this often requires previous practice, and is typically a temporary Sphere. The best physical space is a dedicated room or small separate building that is used for nothing else. A compromise can be made by using a room that is also used for other creative purposes, but deleterious influences such as television should not be allowed in the room during its regular (non-sacromagical) use. Why would you choose work to create the Sphere of Art then undo it with media entertainment that will degenerate the imagination and enervate the life forces [13]?

2: The second zone is the Sphere of Art itself. Within the defined physical location, whatever it may be, the Sphere of Art is built as an energetic construct, within the physical space, and extended partly above and below. This contained but extended Sphere is the second shell, field, or wall, of the overall Vessel.

What is the nature of a shell or wall? It keeps its content safe, focuses whatever is within, and keeps extraneous influences out. All shells or walls, however, have entrances and exits, and we will explore these in terms of the Seven Directions and the Two Sensitive Points.

3: The third zone is the human body. Within the Sphere that is within the physical location, the human body is in the center of the Sphere or at one of the Primary Directions (East, South, West or North). This body-location returns us to manifest Nature, but with the additional understanding that the human body and consciousness-complex is not limited to the Sub-Lunar world, but is a micro-cosmos in itself, capable of mediating the greater Cosmos into the Sub-Lunar realm. We find this concept in the ancient myth of humanity tending the Garden of Eden , with variants in several religions and spiritual traditions.

Working with the Three Zones

We can envision this threefold interaction as three concentric rings, in an idealized model. These three are, as always with two dimensional models, an abbreviation of three concentric spheres. While the room has walls, a roof, and floor, there are no hard boundaries for the two inner spheres, that of the Sphere of Art and the human body. The outer shell or sphere has its (apparently) hard boundary of the physical room as a location for the Sphere of Art. Thus we can envision a pattern of mutually reflecting forces: the first or outer shell, manifest vessel or physical temple, is fully within the Sub-Lunar world of manifest nature; it takes care of itself in many remarkable ways that we take for granted. The second energetic shell can be attuned through conscious adjustment of subtle forces, within the Sphere of Art, and the reflection of both is found in the third component, the human body.

The polarity of the subtle forces is significant at this stage, from Outer to Inner, between the defining physical space and the occupying Sphere, then from Inner to Outer within the consciousness and energy of the human spirit and body interactions.

The Platonic Solids

The interactive patterns generated by the Sphere of Art are those of the famous Platonic Solids, a series of geometric three-dimensional shapes that can be generated within a Sphere. They begin with simple shapes such as the cube and pyramid, but steadily proliferate into increasingly complex polyhedral solids [15].

Well-known in the study of traditional geometry, the Solids are far more than mathematical curiosities. Traditional geometry, as understood by the ancient cultures, is increasingly called "sacred geometry" in recent years...but the truth is that all geometry is sacred, and the simple act of drawing a straight line, a circle, or a point, is a direct theurgic embodiment of cosmic laws of creation and manifestation. A circle drawn consciously in the sand with understanding and interaction is many times more powerful and effective than a complex labyrinth of crystals installed by following a published design or a fashionable trend from a costly seminar or workshop.

The Platonic solids describe and embody inherent cosmic principles of shape and manifestation. Contemporary illustrations of the Tree of Life are flat plans of a three-dimensional conceptual structure that extends further into metaphysical dimensions, though this is seldom understood. The interactions revealed by the Platonic Solids were applied in the building of ancient sacred sites, from sophisticated temples to deceptively simple mounds containing chambers, or stone circles and alignments.

In the early 21st century we are experiencing a remarkable revision of understanding of northern and western European ancient sacred sites. Most recently, new technological advances in archaeology have revealed that the apparently "simple" stone circles of Britain and Ireland were in fact inside complex multiple concentric henges, structures of wooden pillars, often interpreted as being built of massive oak trunks. Thus the persistent notion that these were only crude stone circles is invalidated, and suddenly there is much new work to do in analyzing ancestral sacromagical structures. The principles of sacred geometry and the Platonic Solids are found throughout such ancestral structures, from ancient standing stones to medieval cathedrals, to the pyramids of the Americas and Egypt that have strong connections to Fire Temple spiritual traditions [16].

Shapes and Energies Within a Sphere

Within any sphere, certain significant shapes can be generated through the laws of geometry, and within these shapes, by being present physically, psychically, and spiritually inside them, our consciousness and subtle energies are transformed. This is the wisdom revealed by the Platonic Solids, arising out of the inherent nature of the cosmos.

Much advanced Qabalistic practice consists of visualizing, and interacting with, the Platonic Solids, not on a page, nor as isolated little images, but within a sphere around the practitioner...who is, therefore, *inside the Solids*. The sacred names or letters are, in Hebrew tradition, revealed inscribed upon the faces and angles of the Solids: upon the cube, pyramid, tetrahedron, and so forth. This art is sometimes known as The Cube of Space, and plays a central role in certain aspects of Qabalistic practice. The best known, and most coherent, source text is the *Sefer Yetzirah*, though similar concepts are found scattered throughout Qabalistic literature. *Sefer Yetzirah* works through the sacred qualities of the Hebrew letters and numbers, using them as a language of Creation.

Traditionally the letters of the Hebrew alphabet embody energies, and their hallowed use and powerful glyphic nature represents a lifetime of study and practice. What is seldom stated is that *any set of glyphs* that relates to the Directions and the spiritual qualities may be used, albeit with varying degrees of aptness and aptitude. A number of modern Hermetic Qabalists, most notably W.G. Gray, have attempted to equate the English (Roman) alphabet with the Tree of Life, based on the simple common-sense premise that the language that you speak is the best one for your sacromagical work.

All glyphs, known and unknown as alphabets, can act as an interface for consciousness, and may be "seen" or felt in many dimensions.

In some special practices and traditional initiatory lineages unique alphabets were generated. This principle of glyphic keys is shown in the numerous obscure old texts that have various signs, sigils, and curious alphabets, the meaning of which has been forgotten over the centuries. In some cases they were cryptographic keys, with their meaning only given in verbal teaching. Once the oral tradition is broken, the signs are reproduced by naïve or unscrupulous copyists, who do not have access to the inner meaning. It is best, therefore, to keep modern practice as simple and uncluttered as possible. For an example of a set of *sigils* and *sound-shapes* relating to the Tree of Life and the Directions, see *The Spiritual Dimensions of Music* [17]. These sigils and sound-shapes can be used sparingly within the Sphere of Art, though all normal speech or conversation should be avoided, and the Practice done in Silence.

Creating the Cosmos

When we open, seal, and then empty the Sphere of Art, we are creating a miniature cosmos. After creating the miniature cosmos of the Sphere, we return it to its primal Void, through the Stillness practice within the Sphere. This allows profound telluric and stellar forces to manifest unhindered by the raveling field of the Sub-Lunar realm. Such transformative forces are, so to speak, *invited* by our opening, sealing, and emptying of the Sphere. The oft-published notion of "commanding" spiritual forces is not used, and can be disposed of as both illusory and immature.

Less is Always More

At this stage, the student who has researched the Platonic Solids, the Cube of Space, and the prolix riches of *Sefer Yetzirah* may be over-laden, worried at the potential complexity of the reiterated and interleaved shapes proposed as meditative visualized or theurgic tools and emblems. Here is good news: within the cosmos of the Sphere of Art, the inherent shapes of the Platonic Solids will be spontaneously generated by the subtle energies, *whether we envision them or not*.

In our primary Sphere of Art practice, we build a simple sphere, attuning to the Four Directions and the Sensitive Points above and below. After this building, the Sphere is emptied and made Void. *No more is necessary*, though this, in itself, can be a lifetime spiritual practice. What manifests in the Void is the New Sun, a stellar spiritual power that is free of Sub-Lunar influence, and is born by the fusion of the Earth Light within the planet with a Stellar energy from the cosmos.

The two lights enter through the Two Sensitive Points of Below and Above. Both lights are stellar; one telluric, one astral. Here "astral" is used in its original sense, meaning *of the starry heavens*, not in the popular sense often found today that broadly refers to psychic dimensions of the Sub-Lunar realm. The shifting sense of this vital definition, which has been trivialized in modern use, is discussed in Volume One.

Using the Tree of Life, or Not?

In all of the above, the Tree of Life need not be used at all! Indeed, we might understand that the standard Tree, really one of many representations, though most of the others have faded out of modern publication, shows the Solar System as an interface with the greater cosmos. The standard Tree is a remarkable yet simple model based on what a human sees while standing upon the Earth, the Kingdom. It shows the steady movement, off-planet, from Earth to Moon to Sun and Planets, to Stars. Humanity has always lived within this enfoldment of Three Worlds or nested spheres, Lunar, Solar, and Stellar. A standard or basic Tree of Life illustration is drawn according to our Sub-Lunar conception of the relationship between the Emanations, as follows:

Body (10, Earth), to
Generative Forces (9, Moon, Foundation), to
Thought (8, Mercury, Glory), to
Emotion (7, Venus, Victory), to
Spiritual Entity (6, Sun, Beauty),
and beyond into the higher octaves of
Purification (5, Mars, Severity)
Regeneration (4, Jupiter, Mercy)
Reception (3, Saturn, Understanding)
Emission (2 Neptune or Zodiac, Wisdom) and
Being (1, Uranus, Spirit, *Primum Mobile* or Crown of the Tree).

When we seal the Sphere and empty it, this concept of the Tree is both immediately and progressively rendered Void. Thus we can work fully in the Sphere without an *explicit* Tree of Life, but the Tree itself is *implicit* in the Sealed Sphere, by nature of the

Directions and the Geometric shapes of the Platonic Solids that are generated and empowered.

In *Aesch Mezareph* practice, the Void is filled by the stellar Purifying Fire. Any subsequent actions, physical alchemical, or metaphysical, are commenced from this place of emptiness.

The Tree of Life known in general publication and illustration is a key glyph that resonates within the Platonic Solids. Upon paper it is a two dimensional (flat) convenience map...but it represents three dimensions of space, as with many technical drawings from the past. It is seldom understood that the history of Qabalistic texts in print or indeed inscribed by hand, is strongly defined by the medium of the page, sheet, or surface. From philosophic concepts drawn in the sand, to complex glyphs upon parchment or paper, the early metaphysicians were obliged to find ways to represent multi-dimensional or just three dimensional truths, upon a relatively flat surface.

Beyond the basic three dimensions of fundamental geometry, the Tree of Life embodies metaphysical dimensions that intersect those of the manifest cosmos. This concept is represented by the re-iterative or nested diagrams that show multiple Trees of Life within one another. (Two of my original diagrams, from the 1970's are shown in Figures Thirty Two and Thirty Three).

Remember that these special maps are simultaneously working definitions that help us in our spiritual endeavors, and actual descriptions of territory, both physical and metaphysical, handed down to us in the perennial spiritual traditions. *Self-iteration is a property of the cosmos, not an intellectual idea unique to the functions of the human brain. Harmonious nested iterations are not toys on a computer screen, but properties of number, of geometry, of the mystery of Creation.*

What Tree of Life may be Aligned Within the Sphere of Art?

A large-scale answer to this question could involve the entire Tree of Life, and in detailed practice, the complete tree is mirrored within each individual Emanation in an infinite self-iterating pattern, as is shown in fractal images.

We can, if we choose to do so, work primarily with the classic Tree, reaching from Earth through Moon and Sun to Stars and back again. This is best described as the Solar System Tree, the result of millenniums of observation of the movements, and experience of the subtle forces, generated by the dance of relationship between the Sun and Planets. There are a number of ways in which this simple Solar System Tree of Life, with ten Emanations, may be aligned within the Sphere of Art, and exploring these possibilities bears much fruit in meditation. As always, this should first be a meditative exercise, and never merely limited to pen and paper. Personal notes and drawings, if used at all, are best made *after* meditation or contemplation, after spiritual perception has arisen, otherwise there is a risk that they become empty mental exercises. There is a well-known minor malaise in esoteric students, whereby they spend many hours with pen and paper or with multiple books, but do little or no practical work.

The Tree of Life has multiple iterations, many subtle interactions of the Tree within each Emanation. Thus, there is a complete Tree in each of the Ten Emanations. This interaction can be taken further, for each Path is also a Tree. The Tree of Life is a holism, and is self-iterating, like fractal images, whereby every part has the whole within it, no matter how much you may close in on the details. An excellent short book on this significant fractal nature of the Tree of Life is *The Anatomy of the Body of God* by Frater Achad, wherein he describes the nested Trees and their relationship to Platonic Solids. This book was written before computers and the subsequent calculation of fractal images appeared, and is one of the more interesting, albeit little known, modern classics of original meditation on the nature of the Tree of Life, all the more intriguing as the author states, somewhat obliquely, that he received it from Inner Contacts [18].

Words of Caution and of Liberation

At this point, some words of caution, and of liberation! The Tree embodies and maps a cosmos that ceaselessly proliferates, and the human mind contains inherent seeds of that proliferation.

If we follow the multitude of paths and possibilities mentally, intellectually, we can become stranded or imprisoned in one of the classic spiritual traps. You cannot remain in the mind, the 8th Emanation, forever, no matter how interesting or *scintillating* it may be. Having uttered that caution, we can proceed further with the question of the relationship of the Tree of Life to the Sphere of Art, if such a relationship is necessary in our practices.

The OverWorld and UnderWorld Trees

The Sphere of Art includes a complete Tree of Life, all Ten Emanations of the OverWorld cosmos, and, most important to our modern revival of the art, the reflections or resonances of the Emanations within the body of planet Earth: the UnderWorld Tree. It is, in essence, a 19 Emanation Tree of Life, where the 10th (Kingdom) of the standard Tree is also the 1st (Crown) of the UnderWorld Tree or Roots within the planet. Numerically this Nineteen Emanation Tree resolves back to 10....1+9= 10. In this manner the decimal cycle of the Tree holds good. This pattern is shown in Figure Fifteen (The OverWorld and UnderWorld Tree).

Using the UnderWorld Tree makes a significant difference between Sphere of Art practices and popular or basic modern Qabalistic practices found in general publication. The UnderWorld Tree is an active foundation (note the term Foundation) for the OverWorld Tree, comprising its essential roots, without which nothing will grow.

The Evolution of Metals

When we carefully consider and meditate upon this dynamic of the vital roots of the Tree of Life within the planet, it seems unlikely that the OverWorld Sun in the cosmos owes its existence to roots of metallic gold within the Earth, so the esoteric teaching is about something more subtle.

Both OverWorld and UnderWorld Suns are stellar entities, the Star fragment within the Earth resonating strongly with the OverWorld Sun. It is this resonance, in alchemical tradition, that causes the metals to arise and evolve, hence their emblems in the UnderWorld or alchemical Tree. In the physical sense, the telluric volcanic processes of enormous heat and pressure create and transform the physical elements and metals, and this is mirrored in both physical and spiritual Alchemy.

The classic sequence is:
10 (Carbon or Lava for planetary Earth)
9 Silver for Moon
8 Quicksilver for Mercury
7 Copper for Venus
6 Gold for Sun
5 Iron for Mars
4 Tin for Jupiter
3 Lead for Saturn, plus
2 Salt(s) for Neptune, and
1 Crystal or Sulfur for Uranus.

The UnderWorld Tree is the Foundation of our human growth upon the Tree of Life, it provides our roots and nourishment when we have, as we all do, physical bodies manifest in the Sub-Lunar world. This transformative nourishment within us derives from the same energy that evolves the metals deep within the Earth. It is the mysterious, and still unknown undefined power, that enables a tiny seed to grow and become a flourishing tree.

The alchemists preserved a wisdom tradition that the metals are gradually transformed by this generative power, and that they may evolve. *While our contemporary sciences can analyze increasingly minute stages of the process, the source and nature of the generative power that causes a seed to grow is still mysterious. When the metals are brought to the surface, their natural slow transformation, traditionally likened to that of a seed, enabled through the vitalizing power of the Earth Light, rapidly ceases.* The "metallic seed" is referred to in the *Aesch Mezareph* text, as discussed in Chapter Seven.

Thus, according to this esoteric teaching, mining of precious ores is the equivalent of pulling up a plant, or cutting it off from its roots, whereby it can grow and transform no further. The subtle energies are re-stimulated in the alchemical laboratory. There are many implications to this that can be explored in meditation, with regard to the metals themselves, and to the human role in planetary evolution.

As folkloric tradition reminds us, in the Faery realm of the UnderWorld there is no light of Sun or Moon, but only Starlight. The plant world requires the light of Sun and Moon, the mineral world does not, but is bathed in the invisible Earth Light, the telluric Starlight from the core of the planet. It seems likely, according to contemporary physics, that certain stellar forces also penetrate deeply into the mantle of the Earth, implying direct paths from the starry cosmos into the center of our planet.

A significant meditation can be built upon the role of humanity in the movement of the metals and elements from within the Earth to the surface, in various processes of transformation. This role, with distinct historical and cultural phases, is especially crucial today in our use of nuclear physics; based on highly refined and complex intellectual science without accompanying ethics or spiritual understanding.

The UnderWorld stellar energy, manifesting physically as the active fiery core of our planet, catalyzes the minerals, metals, and elements within our bodies. This is one aspect of the secret Transformation of the Blood that is often hinted at, though seldom revealed. Indeed, at this time it is the most important aspect, because it has been forgotten or repudiated, and is often left out of the mix when initiatory practices are taught or experienced. If a component is left out, the result is either ineffectual or partial.

Energizing and Emptying the Sphere

When we open the Sphere of Art, a major part of our sacromagical task inside the Sphere is un-making its usual mix of contents, and thus to approach Empty. This is done by inviting the Four Archangels to seal and empty the Sphere in its entirety. Our part is to still our own interactions, within ourselves, dissolving our connection to Time, Space, and Movement, and to be conscious of the Two Sensitive Points of above and below. This practice is described in full in Volume One.

The philosophical or metaphysical question of "what Emanations are we working with?" opens out some of the fine details of working within the Sphere. Consider that there is an entire OverWorld Tree of Life, from the Crown of the Sphere, the Sensitive Point above, to the flat plane or mid-plane of the hemisphere (the floor): in a model envisioned in meditation, the 10th Emanation or Kingdom will be half above ground level and half below. Consider that there is an entire UnderWorld Tree from the mid-plane, the floor, down to the Sensitive Point below, with its 1st Emanation or Crown being co-existent with the 10th Emanation, as described above, half above and half below the ground or floor level.

In the standard Tree within the upper hemisphere of the Sphere of Art, the Lunar or Foundation Emanation is emptied; not only the Moon, but the Triple Vessel of Exaltation (Victory/Venus), Scintillation (Glory, Mercury) and Foundation (Moon), as shown in Figure Nine (The Three Vessels). Think of this Triad as a Chalice that is emptied: this is what we do, as humans, when we still Time Space and Movement. We reduce our mental and emotional activity, and further reduce our interactions with the outer world.

The Archangelic forces work to empty the Vessel in terms of subtle forces that appear to be external to ourselves, yet which have a huge interplay in all our magical work. This is a close-up view of the emptying of the Sub-Lunar forces from within the Sphere of Art, something that we seldom explore in detail that will work even if we are not fully aware of it. If you are uncertain about the complexities, work only with the simplicities: Open the Sphere, make it Still, work with the Archangels, and between Above and Below, be Still again and Wait.

An empty Cup alone can fill
With perfect Love,
Be What You Will. (From a ritual text by W.G. Gray, 1960's)

The powerful ritual and meditational concept of Emptying, known in various forms, runs through many esoteric transubstantiation rituals. It brings us back to the idea of the *tohu* that has perhaps its most famous exposition in Lurianic Kabbalah, deriving from earlier root sources. This concept is declared at the opening of *Aesch Mezareph: Elisha was a most notable prophet, an example of natural wisdom, a despiser of riches... For so the true physician of impure metals hath not an outward show of riches, but is rather like the Tohu of the first Nature, empty and void. Which word is of equal number with the word Elisha, viz., 411.*

The process is likened to that of a physician; it is a healing process, transforming the impure metals. The reference to Elisha, and his name being "of equal number", 411, to the *Tohu* of the first Nature is a rich source of insight and tradition. Elisha and Elijah are the two famous fire prophets. By citing Elisha, and his healing of Naaman the leper, the anonymous author invokes a prophetic fire and healing tradition, but expects us to understand that the context is spiritual and alchemical. Not only Elisha/Elijah as historical prophets, are referred to, but the spiritual lineage that they embody. Chapter Seven contains a detailed elucidation of many of the implications in the first chapter of *Aesch Mezareph*.

Only by making our sphere empty can it be filled with the true riches of spirit. Such a philosophical statement has broad applications, and has often been subtly propagandized, but in the Sphere of Art it becomes a focused and precise operation, enabling definable results in terms of transformation. *To make gold you must first have gold* is a classic alchemical aphorism. Two kinds of gold are here referred to: the first may, under certain circumstances, be the common idea of gold as a valuable metal, while the second is the spirit of gold, which is generated by the Sun in the UnderWorld, the Star in the body of Earth, and by your own spiritual origins within your body.

In *Aesch Mezareph* various Qabalistic sources or traditional references are quoted to the effect that there is a subtle process whereby Wisdom can be achieved and this is "substituted" for gold, as material gold without wisdom is of no value. Rather than deliver manifest gold, the Qabalistic methods of *Aesch Mezareph (the Purifying Fire of the crucible)* deliver the means whereby an inner wisdom is achieved; thereafter it becomes the means whereby gold can be made manifest. This dynamic involves a specific relationship between the Directions, and a specific *turning about* of the Directions through human sacromagical or alchemical efforts.

The spirit of gold, the Sun in the UnderWorld, is a stellar energy that fuses the subtle forces and substances of Earth and Stars; it is manifest to us in the OverWorld through the Sun of the Solar System, but is, in the greater sense, the principle of stellar focus, the centrality or harmony inherent in the Stars within their attendant organs or Planets. This spirit of gold is the universal quality of Beauty or Harmony, a stabilizing balance between destruction and creation, or Severity and Mercy. Such polarized forces make up the fabric of the universe, but we can understand them primarily in the context of our own Solar System, the place where we live.

In Chapter Six we will explore an alternative model that demonstrates the processes of Emanation, Elevation, and Transformation, through the use of Purifying Fire.

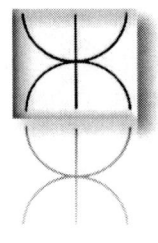

CHAPTER SIX

Chaos Eros and Cosmos

In the Beginning

Another way of understanding the fire energy, *Aesch Mezareph,* is through an ancient classical model, and there is little doubt that many of the basic concepts found in Qabalistic and Hermetic philosophy have roots in ancient Greece, Persia, Sumeria, and Egypt, especially in Pythagorean, Platonic, neo-Platonic, and early astrological systems. In ancient Greek magic and metaphysics, everything was underpinned by the concepts of Cosmos and Chaos.

Today, in our current revival of spiritual traditions and exploratory sacromagical training, the relationship between Chaos and Cosmos defines parameters, and could be said to frame all ways of working. In some ancient sources, the first power appearing from Chaos is Eros, not the Eros of popular entertainment, but a universal Eros, described as the primal *movement* of originative energy from Chaos to Cosmos, eventually creating and commanding even the gods themselves. This divine Eros is a far cry from a chubby cherub wielding a bow or a suggestive pole-dance in a night-club.

When we refer to Eros, it is helpful to remember that there are two forms of Eros in Greek mythology. The first is Movement, often equated with Desire; this Eros was the first movement out of Chaos. The second Eros is said to be the son of Aphrodite and Ares, the brother of Deimos and Phobos and, as in many legends and allegories, the consort of Psyche. We can see that the second Eros is a derivative or lower octave of the first Eros...from an abstract concept of primal movement from Chaos to Cosmos, to the offspring of Love and Conflict (Aphrodite and Ares), brother to Fear and Terror (Deimos and Phobos) that arouses Psyche, or the malleable Soul.

Eros, the power that *moves,* is essential to successful rituals, be they social or sacred. Eros includes human sexuality, but is greater than personal gratification. When we work to elevate the metals or substances, and their sparks within ourselves, within the Sphere of Art, there is a continual interchange of energies, steadily accelerating and building to peak of intensity as ascend the Tree of Life. This is, of course, reminiscent of the sexual act...not because physical sexuality reigns supreme, but because the divine Eros is the moving force behind all exchanges, from the most minute to the exaltation of Stars. Eros is the driving power behind the mysterious Laws of magic and theurgy, hence all magic could be, paradoxically, called "sex magic", bearing in mind that human gratification through physical sex is the biological outlet for much deeper spiritual forces. *I am fixed and I am free* is one of the assertions of an ancient mystery ritual, declaring the relationship between movement (freedom) and essential containment of such movement (fixedness).

If we can discover how to work with this interaction, all physics and metaphysics is, potentially, at our disposal. The secret has always been that we should allow whatever is already present to be itself, rather than seek to enforce nature to conform to our desire for profit. By corrupting and polluting the natural world we destroy ourselves. By discovering the inherent interactions and polarities, moved by Eros, be it through science or spiritual perception, and thereby honoring the world in which we live, we come into a deeper relationship not only with the planet, but with the cosmos that is mirrored in our Earth and Solar System.

The Laws of Magic and the Sphere of Art

What we think of as the laws of magic are the binding forces of the cosmos that enable function, generated by the relationship of the Four Root Elements of Air, Fire, Water, and Earth. The late W.G. Gray, wrote in the 1960's that people always take elemental laws for granted, certain that fire will not rage out of the faucet, or water pour from electrical outlets [34]. This deceptively simplistic example is invaluable in meditation. Our entire machine-based culture thrives on such unconsidered expectations that everything will continue to work for us. For practical purposes, nowadays defined by physics, machinery will probably work as expected, most of the time. Can this semi-certainty also apply to the laws of magic? How do such laws, if discovered, apply within the Sphere of Art? Is there, perhaps, a greater certainty to be discovered? Another mentor, the late A. R. Heaver (1900-190), who I have termed the Hidden Glastonbury Adept, repeatedly taught that what we need is not more Power, but further Purification. This is also an Elemental teaching, but in the higher octaves, relating to the transformative fire of *Aesch Mezareph*, that is also Eros.

If we are truly to attempt to discover and understand the Laws of Magic, we should begin with the laws of Cosmos and Chaos that we have begun to observe and re-discover in our universe since Frederick Herschel (1738-1822) and his sister Caroline (1750-1848) produced the first modern mirror-lensed telescopes in the 18th century. We can think of this as rediscovery, without in any way diminishing the stunning effect of Herschel's discoveries, because there is considerable evidence that the ancient cultures understood many aspects of cosmology, presumably without telescopes. Such knowledge was suppressed in much of Europe, and later forgotten, due to the dominant influence of the Roman Church, until the Renaissance period took a fresh look at the fragments of ancient wisdom remaining. While the discovery of the true nature of Stars and comets in the 18th and 19th century punched deeply into the absurdity of Christian dogma, it confirmed the teachings of the perennial esoteric traditions, for they have always described a greater cosmos beyond the delusion or propaganda regarding a vengeful creator god.

The Laws of Magic are the Laws of Cosmos, but they frequently act in what are, for us, uncomfortable ways; the planetary elemental powers of weather, earthquakes, and volcanic eruptions have recently come to the foreground of our attention due to a chain of events in the early 21st century. Yet, far from being chaotic, these vast upheavals follow natural laws of the Elements within planet Earth, mirroring those of the Cosmos.

Human evolution is supposedly accelerating, yet we are nothing in comparison to cosmic activity, where infinite clouds of Stars are born and raging Planets are hurled out into orbit. The true power of Eros is the power that births Star-fire. We just tag along, miserably reducing Eros to our self-focused little human sexual scenarios. What is thought of as "destructive" here on Earth is often an aspect of long-term laws of creation. So typical definitions of Law or Cosmos, and originative Chaos, are subjective and are mainly human-centric. We are indeed the center of our human lives, and this has to be a valid starting point. A rigid center can only decay and collapse. Our center must have flexibility, and potential for adaptive transformation.

Through magic, theurgy and thaumaturgy, we can find new centers, and we desperately need, as a collective, to grasp the truth, to know that humans are not the rulers of planet Earth, but are ephemeral beings clinging precariously on to her fringes. Typically this realization leads to discomfort, and we often take refuge in escapist religion. There are two paths toward a solution: one takes us off-planet the other takes us in-planet. On both paths the driving power is the divine Eros, polarized as the Evolutionary and Involutionary Streams, the Red and White Dragons of Bardic Tradition. To be in balance, we need to have traveled both paths, ideally in one lifetime.

If There Are Hidden Laws, What Are They Hiding From?

In the popular revival of interest in magic there are many interpretations of "magical laws". Overall, the subject is extremely confused and ill-represented, mainly due to commercialization and endless copying in publication. Nevertheless, progress has been made during the 20th century toward clarification, and, as is often the case, we are finding that a return to some simple yet potent practices brings us back to earlier spiritual roots.

In general magical arts, rituals are often said to take advantage of hidden laws, yet are also said to obviate or by-pass such laws. When a magical circle is cast or opened, it is a miniature cosmos, wherein ritualists formulate how cosmic laws might operate.

Typically this mini-cosmos is arranged according to traditional patterns of elements, seasons, deities, spiritual allies, and so forth. This is a helpful idea, as it reminds everyone that arbitrary laws may not always be applicable, and that it may be best to work with what is already present rather than declare that you are opting out of the cosmos in a petulant manner and then be disappointed that your ritual did not go anywhere.

Magic, from primal ancestral traditions to the most abstract esoteric practices, works with existing laws that underpin the greater cosmos. Both theurgy and thaumaturgy respect and attune to such laws. The Sphere of Art takes this classic process one stage further, and affirms that the circle is truly an emblem for a sphere. No entities, no gods and goddesses or others, are invoked into the Sphere of Art, but powerful spiritual presences embrace it and protect it, according to certain hidden laws that can be proven through experience. Faith and religion are irrelevant in the Sphere of Art: it proves itself through Stillness and subsequent experience.

In old–fashioned language we would say that the Four Archangels wrap their six-fold wings around the Sphere, and remove all Sub-Lunar content from it, through their inherent role and power as Guardians. This occurs in an "automatic" manner, by the very nature of the Archangels, rather than through invocation, evocation, or the childish notion of commanding potent spiritual beings.

Thus the standard magical circle, or micro-cosmos, has components of elements, directions, gods and goddesses, and spiritual allies, *because they are known to work*. Their interactions are due to the power of Eros moving between the supernal conditions of Chaos and Cosmos, and further Polarizing as shown on the Tree of Life. Such a movement or wave pattern generates long-enduring resonances that we conceive of as laws, and in turn these enable the forming of entities, gods, goddesses, spirits, humans, teapots, prawns, elephants, asteroids, and, most significant in our sacromagical work, Archangels and angels, though not necessarily in the order listed.

Thus a harmonious mini-cosmos can be attuned inside the Sphere of Art, which is the next level of working beyond the more popular magical circle. This mini-cosmos acts like an engine, a containing vessel for energy, but rather than burning irreplaceable fossil fuel to drive a shaft, the magical engine utilizes the inexhaustible Roots of Creation, the Elements, according to the way that they work already.

It is much easier to work with those cosmic forces that are already present, than to fight them. Such a magical engine may seem, to those who do not understand it, to work wonders, but it is in harmony with the laws, all the way back to the primal cause of Being. This requires effort and endurance. A helpful precept for meditation and for sacromagical disciplines is this: *it takes a long time to make something happen instantly by magic.* Yet this is no different to other skills; musical training can take years of patient practice and theory, but the great performance flows unhindered to inspire the audience.

Undo What You Will

Often ritualists have been, and will continue to be, frustrated when their commands, wishes, and invocations seem to have no results. Let's be honest over this issue, for many have experienced it. Those who get frustrated with the popular methods of easy-sale magic and subsequently give up, soon return to living within the unconscious field of everyday life, knowing that water will not issue from the electrical outlets (except perhaps in California during a wet winter). Those who do not give up will still be repeatedly frustrated, but will steadily grow beyond egocentric reaction, discovering that the laws of Cosmos, driven by Eros, will often trump our somewhat minor human ritual expectations.

Magicians, theurgists, and mystics of all traditions, have long since learned to align with potent laws, and to use them creatively and imaginatively.

Before you can move ahead with such a choice, you must decide what you want to *undo* in yourself, to discover what must be given up, to be free. The secret, if it is a secret at all, is that you must build a dialogue with the consciousness and energy of the seemingly mysterious cosmic laws, benefiting from them by participating in them. There is a soft boundary in all magic between Energy and Entity, which is why rituals have always involved both human and spirit beings. Through dialogue with Entities, you enable an interaction with Energies. Energies, Entities, and Eros, are the triad of practical sacromagical methods. This triad is a mirror image of the greater triad of Chaos Cosmos and Eros, with Eros linking both triads, as shown in Figure Sixteen, (Chaos, Cosmos, and Eros).

In working with the Sphere of Art this fundamental principle of theurgic magic is applied, so to speak, in reverse. We aim to empty the Sphere, and ourselves, and cease all invocations, awaiting a New Sun to arise out of the spiritual fusion of stellar and telluric energies in the center. Yet this is also Eros, descending, ascending, and fusing into a bright pure Star.

Is Chaos Untidy?

Nowadays in general use the word "chaos", typically means something messy, conflicted, random, turbulent, and without order. In ancient Hebrew the first primal cause of creation is called "tohu". This *tohu* (the term appears in the Torah, Old Testament, and in mystical Qabalistic and alchemical texts) is the source of all worlds, moving out of the Void or Chaos, and gradually taking form, pattern, and relationship as the Cosmos. Its innate impulse to *move* is what the Greeks called Eros, whom even the gods and goddesses must obey. If you speak modern Hebrew, however, the same word, *tohu*, is used to mean untidy, as in a mother's comments on the discordant mess of her teenager's bedroom. This is typical of our movement away from a spiritual and magical understanding toward a material one, yet it still holds hidden meaning. All movement arises from Eros, including movement toward ignorance and materialism.

Chaos is not untidy...it is *pre-tidy*. Chaos is the unformed *force* from which *form* comes into manifestation. Some popularized schools of magic have suggested that chaotic forces can be invoked, by-passing greater cosmic laws, side-stepping the laws of nature, to gain rapid results. Approaches to this perspective, found in both publication and practice, vary from wise and profound to foolish and shallow. Any form of spiritual practice or magic that inflates the ego of the practitioner is potentially very dangerous indeed, for it traps him or her in the solipsistic map, and ensures that the real territory is lost to perception and understanding. Perhaps the most pernicious New Age dogma is "I create my own reality".

Fission or Fusion from Chaos

The primary example of chaos or by-pass magic, devoid of ethical considerations, is nuclear fission. By unbinding the laws of form and manifestation that prevail upon planet Earth, a terrible destructive energy is unleashed, something so inimical that it has a further long-term degenerative effect upon all life forms that absorb its deadly radiation over thousands of years. So within the idea of chaos magic, everyone should think deeply upon their own inner Reactors ...are they frustrated with what seem to be restrictive laws, or are their rituals reaching into the hidden primal chaos, drawing upon the pre-tidy that enables the paradoxically tidy? Little wonder that the most dangerous structures made by humanity are reactors, be they in a bomb or in a power station.

Eros unleashed in an inappropriate way will destroy, but Eros moving with grace and harmony will bless and enlighten. This is the difference between fission and fusion: as in physics, so in metaphysics. The sacromagical tradition of the "Kings of Edom", referred to in *Aesch Mezareph* holds the key to understanding, and is explored in the next chapter.

To Counter the Threat of Nuclear Armageddon

One of the stated aims of the first Sanctuary of Avalon, founded by A R Heaver and Polly Woods in the 1950's was "to counter the threat of nuclear Armageddon". By which they meant we should seek to open ourselves, and therefore our world, to spiritual forces and Inner Contacts of harmonious *fusion*, as the only true counterbalance to destructive fission. In spiritual mediation within the new Sanctuary of Avalon on the slopes of Glastonbury Tor and its counterparts in the USA, this dedicated attunement is still active today [7]. Stillness, Sphere of Art, and *Aesch Mezareph* practices are the only practices within the Sanctuary, which is a Sanctuary of Silence.

Evil as Energy

No one can think for long about Law and Chaos, Cosmos and Eros, without being confronted by the idea of evil. Modernist culture is dominated by unhealthy ideas of evil; in the entertainment industry many definitions of evil are nothing more than ephemeral grotesque stereotypes. What is bad to one culture may seem good and desirable to another, and definitions of evil change from land to land, race to race, religion to religion, and from century to century.

Politicians may talk about the greater good, but people seldom see it being respected. Mostly one culture tries to impose its "good" upon the "evil" of other cultures. History shows this pattern repeatedly, right into the present day. Current international conflicts may indeed seem to be about barely disguised appropriation of oil or mineral reserves and gas pipelines, but at another level, barely below the surface, they are truly wars over differing definitions of evil, arising from deeply entrenched dogmatic religions.

On a larger scale, natural destructive forces are often type-cast as "evil", while natural creative forces are "good". Such simplistic dualism is found in many religions, and is often successfully propagandized; it is really a superficial formulation of the deeper ideas of Cosmos and Chaos. Anything that follows Cosmic law but is fearsome, such as an erupting volcano, is supposedly evidence of inimical forces, or even the wrath of a deity. But it is, in truth, nothing more than energy at work according to cosmic law on Earth. The only "evil" or "punishment for evil" relative to natural events is within the mind, due to ignorance, innocence, or propaganda. The late Dion Fortune (1890-1946), who had a substantial influence on the revival of magic in the early 20th century, proposed that evil was nothing more nor less than misplaced energy. The effect of destructive energy is often relative to wherever people would prefer the energy to be, and not truly "evil" in itself.

In Charles Williams' occult novel, *War in Heaven* (1930), there are two black magicians. One is a flamboyant fantasist, indulging in sexual depravity, spite, greed and self-indulgence, while attempting to steal spiritual power from a sacred chalice. The other is a quiet, apparently unassuming man, living modestly as a back-street herbal pharmacist. He invokes polarized forces out of Chaos into an empty room, thereby causing the entire building to vanish when police search for him. Yet, paradoxically, it is this quiet and chilling mediator of "evil" that enables, despite himself, the rescue of the sacred chalice from spiritual perversion thus preventing the sacrifice of an innocent child. There seems to be little doubt that the second character is the real "black" magician, while the first is an immature egocentric poser. The rest I would recommend you read for yourself! The boundary between Cosmos and Chaos is what Williams is really exploring in this story...and it is a soft boundary. Eros crosses to and fro through that boundary, that veil, and anyone can cross with it. Indeed, everyone crosses it many times at each death and rebirth. If we can Still this repeated cycle, even momentarily, we come into the greater consciousness of the territory, and lose the habitual map. This is the aim of all the spiritual traditions of liberation. Not to reject or repudiate Eros, but to discover the hidden ways of Eros, and travel those hidden ways toward poise and stillness beyond interactions, beyond polarities.

Compassion and Coercion

Once you become aware of this soft boundary between Cosmos and Chaos, an ethical path can be chosen, to work magic harmoniously and compassionately, rather than coercively. Through this, the idea of opposites such as good and evil, law and chaos, slowly fades away, and is replaced by a deeper perception of cosmic patterns. To enable such clarity a few significant questions could be voiced, and then taken into meditation. A helpful practice is to meditate on the following questions outside the Sphere of Art, in general meditation, then to meditate upon them again while within the sealed and activated Sphere. The answers may change.

1: What are the cosmic laws that seem to affect you most?

2: How may you truly relate to them rather than feel subject to them?

3: And, perhaps the biggest task of all, how can you build a positive relationship with primal Chaos through spiritual work?

In our context of the Sphere of Art and *Aesch Mezareph* we can find some constructive and concise answers through our sacromagical work. You will, of course, discover your own additional answers to the three questions, but the following suggestions may be helpful.

1: *What are the laws that affect us most?*

The cosmic laws that most obviously affect us most are those that seem negative, at first, and are the most difficult to empty from the Sphere of Art. In standard meditational techniques these are often typified as emotions, desires, impulses and so forth. Stilling these through gently withdrawing from engagement is a standard meditative art. But what are the laws behind such typical patterns? Where is the attraction, where is the repulsion? What Emanation of the Tree of Life will generate the aversions or addictions, and what Emanation will purify them? What metal or substance can be elevated to help us with our understanding of Cosmic laws, of their effect upon us, and on the world in which we live? Here is where the practical work in our preceding chapters will be of great help. Next we might consider those subtle laws that affect us positively...the spiritual forces of blessing that may activate in our lives as a result of dedicated sacromagical and theurgic work. Try to discover what relationship there is between these positive patterns (laws and energies) and any negative ones that you have discerned. Such discernment must be discovered in meditation within the activated Sphere of Art, not solely through self-analysis, intellectual comparisons, or a psycho-therapeutic approach. The Sphere of Art will always amplify and accelerate whatever is offered within it, and this is a law of theurgic magic that you should always remember, as it will reveal much about your inner transformations and re-iterations.

2: How may we truly relate to cosmic laws rather than feel subject to them?

In our typical mapping of the territory of consciousness, from birth to death, we relate to the cosmic laws almost entirely by reaction. Indeed, it is this reaction in the growing field of thought, emotion, and desire, which slowly assembles the map and blots out a clear sense of the original territory. That territory is essentially pure, but its purity may be unbearable for us as humans in our present life. The secret is to work with those laws that steadily and progressively unravel the skeins and threads that are woven into the map, until it thins, becomes transparent, and eventually fades away altogether. Gradually we discover that we can have a *mutual interaction* with certain sacromagical forces and their laws, and the problem of *subjective reaction* gradually fades away.

3: How may we build a positive interaction and relationship with primal Chaos through our magical work?

The answer to this is at once the most significant and the simplest. In an activated and emptied Sphere of Art, embraced by the Archangelic presences, the forces of primal Chaos become transmuted into a new cycle of Cosmos, a pristine Cosmos that we have not previously perceived. This cannot be done without a prior emptying of the Vessel.

Paradoxically Chaos becomes accessible through order, and order through Chaos, for any excess of one will lead to the other in a repeated cycle, until we begin to work in a conscious co-operative relationship with such spiritual forces. Or to put it another way, Mom will make us tidy our Messy Room and we will mess it up again and again until we grow up, and eventually leave the room behind, tidy clean and empty. *Tohu wa bohu.*

The lowest octave of this movement-cycle, this Eros cycle, is illustrated in the tarot trump of the Wheel of Fortune, but there are two further octaves, the Wheels of Justice and of Judgment, that reach deep into the Cosmos. An effective meditation can be made on these three trumps, beginning with Fortune, then Justice, then Judgment. Their interactions upon the Tree of Life are shown in Figure Eight. Fortune rotates between Feelings and Thoughts, founded upon the Lunar realm. Justice, the next octave, rotates between Creation and Destruction, Mercy and Severity, founded upon the Solar realm. Judgment is a supernal wheel, rotating between Wisdom and Understanding. Now that you have an understanding of the Sphere of Art, you will have already perceived that these are not Three Wheels at all...but three nested spheres of Cosmos, progressively emerging from Chaos, empowered by Eros.

Effective transformation is achieved through the prime mover, Eros. When the divine Eros moves, anything can move with it, and the relationship between Chaos and Cosmos becomes interactive, loose, and beautiful. This is the real secret behind the ancient idea of the redemption and uplifting of Nature into Spirit, which is nothing to do with formal religion or presumed salvation, but is a pure matter of Energy, Entity, and Eros, of movement between Chaos and Cosmos.

In our next chapter, the Qabalistic and Alchemical instructions and concepts of the first Chapter of *Aesch Mezareph* are analyzed, and elucidated in terms of the hidden practices of the Fire Temple and the Sphere of Art.

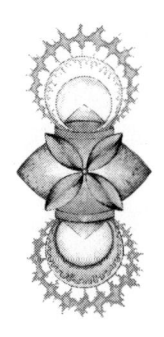

CHAPTER SEVEN

An Elucidation of the First Chapter of:

Aesch-Mezareph, The Purifying Fire.

Preamble

I would like to state, at the outset, that I am fully aware of the vast school of thought and many substantial profound publications, that consider the methods of *Aesch Mezareph* and similar historic books solely as physical experiments, albeit of a hidden science different from that of standard materialism. I have no issue with this, but I am not offering an interpretation of physical Alchemy. My understanding is that the physical and the spiritual may not be separated by artifice, and that the task of the individual is to bring them into perfect unity. Some paths toward this unity focus primarily on spiritual methods, others focus on physical experiment. Ultimately it is the inner condition of the meditator, the alchemist, the Qabalist, that will confirm and establish unity; not the path itself, but the condition arrived at after the long journey.

There is no doubt that a large portion of *Aesch Mezareph* describes technical processes of crucible and furnace, the chemical and alchemical transformations through *subtle graduations of fire.* What is significant is that the physical experiments are only carried out after intensive spiritual preparation, described in the first chapter and continuing through each of the following seven, and that physical processes are inseparable from the spiritual process of refining through the forces of the Emanations [33].

The translation of the first chapter is quoted in full in Appendix Seven. Where the original is quoted below, its spelling is retained, so there are several variant spellings found herein, due to the vagaries of 17th century orthography, and of 19th century interpretations of Hebrew into English.

Qabalistic Origins

As defined in our previous chapters, "Kabbalah" or "Kabala" or any variant, refers to Jewish traditional Kabbalah, while "Qabalah" refers to Hermetic or Neo-Platonic Qabalah. The relationship between the three primary cultural streams of Qabalah/Kabbalah is discussed in *The Miracle Tree* [11]. The inner spiritual tradition that is called by K or Q words is, of course, not culturally or religious owned, but derives from spiritual perception, regardless of language or historical location.

Aesch Mezareph combines Kabbalah and Alchemy and offers several esoteric methods of transformation. While it originally came into shape as a published text before the 17th century when it was first translated into Latin, from a Hebrew or Aramaic original, it seems likely from internal evidence that it began as a set of working notes aphorisms and methods intended for practical verbal elucidation. *Aesch Mezareph* is not a Christian text, there are no New Testament references, and the anonymous original author cites traditional Jewish sources only, such as Torah, Talmud, or Mishnah [19].

References to angels or Archangels are curiously absent, perhaps because they were prohibited in the particular tradition followed by the original author, or, more likely in my opinion, because they formed part of a direct verbal teaching that must have accompanied the original working notes. There are many prohibitions against working with Archangels or angels, usually associated with detailed tables of their names, attributes, powers, and sigils. The perceptive reader can draw his or her own conclusions as to why something noted and later published was supposedly proscribed in practice. Whatever the reasons, the missing angelic attributes are given in our previous chapters and appendices, with special reference to the Sphere of Art practice.

The Translations of *Aesch Mezareph*

The aim of the first translator of *Aesch Mezareph*, Knorr von Rosenroth in the 17th century C.E., rendering Hebrew or Aramaic into Latin, was to bring Jewish and Christian mysticism together, under a Christian unification. *Aesch Mezareph* is only a small part of his much larger work *Kabbala Denudata*, a massive collection of some of the key works of Jewish Kabbalah. We do not, however, see any traces of this aim of Christian unification in *Aesch Mezareph*, so it would seem that there was no dogmatic editing. The entire original Latin and Hebrew text, photographed from an original edition, can be found on-line at the Jewish National University Library [20].

The aim of the second translator, in 1714, working from von Rosenrath's Latin and Hebrew into English, was primarily alchemical, rather than religious. This translator calls himself "Lover of Philalethes", referring to the copious and influential works of Eirenaeus Philalethes, from the 17th century. Philalethes was the pseudonym of a prolific alchemical writer who influenced Newton, Leibnitz, and Locke, among many others. So in both cases, there is at least a fair chance that the text has not been propagandized, no matter how fragmented it became prior to restoration.

The third editor, the remarkable Hermetic scholar and occultist Dr. Wynn W Westcott, (19th century) had both knowledge and practice of Hebrew Kabbalah, and provided insightful notes, some of which are quoted below. Dr. Westcott states that he worked from the pseudonymous 18th century English translation, making corrections according to his knowledge of Hebrew and of the Latin original (Appendix Six).

Humor and Hyper-text

To my mind, there is a thread of humor running through *Aesch Mezareph*, as some of the intentional transpositions of attributes are at times outrageous. Lest there be any doubt, this is, humor or not, an extremely profound text. I hope that my elucidation of

Chapter 1 will show what may be hidden throughout *Aesch Mezareph*. As Chapter 1 is the source and model for the further development of the remaining seven chapters, it greatly assists in our understanding of the entire book. There is no need, whatsoever, to study this elucidation in order to practice the Sphere of Art operations as described in the preceding chapters of this book. Indeed, a deeper understanding of the original *Aesch Mezareph* source text might be found after the Sphere of Art practices have been explored and established.

The entire *Aesch Mezareph* consists of densely allegorical or codified and nested chapters that take the seven metals, plus alchemical sulfur, salt, and mercury, through each of the Ten Emanations, the same process that is described in modern terms, as a Sphere of Art practice, in our preceding chapters. Nor is this an unusual concept to find: the central premise of Qabalistic traditions is that we can work with the Tree of Life to transform ourselves and come into greater communion with the divine Being. The rest, as Rabbi Hillel famously said, is commentary [27]. The commentary that Hillel describes, however, is a unique and hallowed practical guide to ways of living rightly and ethically, not a literary or abstract commentary. On a smaller scale, if providing a commentary on *Aesch Mezareph* (or any other mystical text) serves to enable us to do something effective with our Qabalah, our metals, our inner energies, such a commentary is worth attempting.

There are a number of Biblical references in the text that expand in many directions, leading to other Biblical, Torah, Talmudic or Mishnaic references. These essential and thought provoking references are not offered here in any dogmatic sense, but as fluid allegorical passages with many layers of meaning. Typically references were cited as "authorities" to support a writer's thesis, and while this may well be the case in *Aesch Mezareph*, the references go much further, for they open avenues to many insights and suggestions, creating a hyper-text replete with hidden meaning and practical methods. This method of elucidation, well known in Jewish religious, philosophical, and mystical tradition, is often baffling or even annoying for the contemporary reader who is, inevitably, outside the subtle field of traditional consciousness required to make sense of it all, in addition to lacking the essential scholarship. This short elucidation merely reveals some of the hidden material, which surfaces easily as soon as we reach for it. No doubt there is much more to be revealed, not only in textual analysis, but in direct meditation and through communion with Inner Contacts.

The Original Plan

Aesch Mezareph has eight chapters. The original plan seems to have been that chapter 1 described the cosmic creation mystery through the Three Supernal Emanations, and the seven following chapters reveal Qabalistic and alchemical methods and insights that unfold according the progression of the subsequent Seven Emanations, their embodying Seven Planets, and their Seven Metals. By chapter 7 there is a point where the direction of Emanation has changed, though this is not openly declared. Sometimes we are descending from the Stars to the Earth, while at others we are ascending from Earth to Heaven. Certain elements or substances are found both in the Supernal Emanations and in the world of Nature, especially lead. We will explore this apparent confusion later, and discover its hidden implications.

There are multiple practices hidden with the book, and to disentangle and elucidate the entire text, all eight chapters, would be a major work. Typically, this text, and all others in similar vein, cannot be deciphered unless the interpreter has previous knowledge and experience of both Qabalah and Alchemy, thus proving the famous frustrating paradoxical alchemical adage "to make gold you must first have gold". We should remember, however, that all such texts were considered handbooks to be clarified and activated through initiatory oral tradition and direct teaching, and that they were not intended to be read as training manuals in the modern sense [28].

The Eight Chapters Unfold as Follows:

Chapter I: The Qabalistic and alchemical allegory of Elisha and Naaman. This allegory is found embedded within, and deeply connected to, a description of the relationship between the Emanations/*Sephiroth,* and the Alchemical principles and metals. The most significant aspect of the Elisha story is his relationship to *Tohu*, the Void and the descending River of Wisdom and Understanding, also called Judgment. (Further expounded in A.M. Chapter 7)

Chapter 2: Describes ten forms of gold, relating to the Ten Emanations or *Sephiroth*. The *kamea* or magic square of gold is also given. So-called "magic" squares are reiterative patterns of numbers, offering simple demonstrations of the same principles as modern fractal sets, employing inherent properties of number that show a suggestive coherence and self-iteration. Dr. Westcott notes that the *kamea* given in Chapter 2 is not the true *kamea* for gold, which presumably would have been taught verbally to initiates, and he offers an alternative [25].

Chapter 3. Silver is next related to the Ten *Sephiroth*; we are also offered the *kamea* of silver. Next comes iron, and the transformations of animal forms, with the *kamea* of iron. The animal transformations are of especial interest to the esoteric student.

Chapter 4. Describes tin and Jupiter and the associated *kamea*.

Chapter 5. Describes brass, its tenfold relationship to the Emanations, and its *kamea*.

Chapter 6. Lead and *Chokmah* are said to be related (but this should really be lead and Binah, Saturn). The tenfold elevation and Kamea of lead are given. Chapter 6 continues with a description of *Ariah*, the lion, more of *Naaman*, and the nature of alchemical antimony.

Chapter 7. Describes *Jarden* as the river Jordan, a river of Clear Judgment, Bounty and Rigor.

Also in this chapter *Jesod* is said to be quicksilver or metallic mercury (when it is truly silver), and the mystery of Edomite Wife is partially revealed, along with a further *kamea*.

Chapter 8. Partially reveals the mystery of *Juneh*, the Dove, of *Jarach*, and of the Moon. Lastly *Gophrith*, Sulphur, is discussed.

Each of the metals is taken through a tenfold exposition, while it is primarily related to one specific "home" or root Emanation, such as copper for *Netzach* and Venus, Gold for the Sun and *Tiphareth* and so forth. Its nature in each of the ten Emanations is also obliquely described. Once the text is clarified and re-ordered it reveals the correct order for the process of elevating each of the metals through each of the Ten Emanations, as described in our preceding chapters of practical work within the Sphere of Art. The intentional confusion would not have presented any real challenge to a trained Kabbalist, but would certainly guard the secrets of some of the processes from, say, a curious Christian metallurgist, or one of the followers of the deluded materialist *Gehazi* (disobedient servant of Elisha), of whom we shall hear more shortly.

Depths of Allusion....or Illusion?

It could be argued that an overtly demonstrative and almost but never quite covert and secretive mystical alchemical text is loaded with as many images, references, and mixtures of religious or magical sources as possible. Presumably an author would do this to create an effect, to generate wonder or baffled confusion. This style certainly seems to be more likely, progressively more true, of later occult texts seeking to cash in on the occult revival, and anxious to generate almost meaningful product.

Yet such an argument is an easy prop for cynicism based on lack of scholarship; it does not hold up when an older source, such as a Qabalistic or alchemical text, is examined in depth. Indeed, it would be more accurate to propose that many, but certainly not all, such texts have infinite depths of allusion and multiple enfolded mutually interactive sets of nested meanings. This complexity is at its highest, as is well known, in Hebrew Kabbalah.

Of the many remarkable modern English language books on Kabbalah, perhaps the most comprehensive are those of the late Rabbi Aryeh Kaplan (1935-83) [1].

When we approach an obscure and undoubtedly confused text such as *Aesch Mezareph*, why we might want to dive deeply, or dive at all, into such complexity, is another matter. If it is just curious old junk, and many would argue that it is, we would be better employed in simple meditation. If it contains the remnants of an enduring system of inner transformation, then may be worth some effort.

My understanding is that any exploration of historic texts must be combined with practical work in meditation, theurgy, or sacromagical disciplines and arts. Dive deep, but keep a vessel for navigation. Intellect alone, (8th Emanation, Mercury) is an appropriate vessel for Inspiration (1st Emanation, Crown, Uranus) only when it is used with Rigor (5th Emanation, Severity, Mars). It is easy to let the questing intellect become dazzled by the Splendor and Brilliance (8th Emanation) of all the myriad interconnections in Qabalistic and Alchemical texts. If this mercurial ferment begins, you may become lost, endlessly mistaking a flurry of incomplete maps for insights into the actual territory.

The late W.G. Gray, who frequently employed effectively simple mechanistic models for spiritual teaching, compared this process to extending the Tree of Life sideways, outwards to the left, from the 8th Emanation alone, thus bringing a tilt of imbalance. He made a demonstration model out of small rubber balls of equal size and weight joined by cocktail sticks, and, sure enough, it fell over. While this seemed eminently silly to me, at the age of 23, nowadays I can recognize it as a very old form of teaching, for the properties of the material world (the balls and sticks) derive from the properties of the spiritual world, *and are not separate from them*. This is, of course, the repeated message in *Aesch Mezareph*.

Texts employing Qabalistic style are extremely dense and rich in cross-references and hyper-references. Such a text is *Aesch Mezareph* or *Purifying Fire*. Cryptic allusions and annotated cross-references often guide us to other texts, and we find many examples of this in *Aesch Mezareph*; such examples can be read and meditated upon, and the relationships between the references and the original text frequently include hyper-references. I would hazard that you could spend your whole life working with this one short book of eight chapters, and it would not be a wasted life! It requires an ethical stance, discipline, compassion, and detachment from selfish materialism. These qualities, through the practical methods described, gradually become the spring-boards for deeper understanding and wisdom.

Hyper-references can usually only be understood if the reader is within the initiatory or mystical tradition that is at the root of the main text, though some appear to be nothing more than simple puns. This is especially complex in Hebrew or any other multi-level language.

Other remarkable examples include, but are by no means limited to, old Irish or Welsh, as is evidenced by the early manuscripts remaining to us from the poets and bards. In both old Hebrew and old Irish, for example, it was possible to say at least three things simultaneously in one text…having what appears to be a main narrative, true unto itself, that carries at least two further stories or sequences, sometimes of completely different meaning. In old Irish, Welsh, and Hebrew, single words or short phrases, specifically located in a verse or sentence, can convey further hidden meaning. This multifold concept is especially alien to the modern mind, which has been bludgeoned into simplistic literalism through the dregs of scientific method trickling down into our woeful education system.

The tradition of an openly hidden meaning is especially significant in the numeration of Hebrew words, for each letter is also a number, and their numerical values can be totaled, thus defining a new word. This art of *gematria* is found in many places in our text, such as the connection between the word *tohu* and the name *Elisha* that opens the chapter, and upon which the entire text rests as a foundation. We will return to this shortly.

In an English translation we are somewhat limited by the language, and in the case of *Aesch Mezareph*, the Hebrew or

Aramaic original seems to be lost, so the text has already moved from Hebrew to Latin, then to English. We must, therefore, live with the translations that we have, until either an original manuscript is discovered, or a better translation can be made of the 17th century Knorr von Rosenroth Latin and Hebrew text.

There is no claim here, in this short elucidation, to being academic, or rigorous beyond the contextual focus and insights that are offered regarding the hidden practices within the source text. The reader will discover how rich and multi-leveled the original text is from our basic expansion of the first chapter. There is little doubt that delving into Hebrew would produce many further allusions and hyper-references, but such a major task is beyond the scope of this book, which aims to offer practical methods over academic or linguistic references.

From this point onwards, the text of *Aesch Mezareph* is quoted in short sections, with elucidation commentary and references. Further chapters are referred to as A.M. 1, A.M. 2, and so forth.

Elisha and the Fire Temple Tradition

Elisha was a most notable prophet, an example of natural wisdom, a despiser of riches, as the history of the healing of Naaman shows, (2 Kings, c.5, v.16) and (Elisha was) therefore truly rich.

The key words here are Elisha, prophet, natural wisdom, riches, and healing. Both Elisha and his master Elijah were fire prophets, embodying an ancient sacred fire tradition. The story in the Old Testament wherein Elijah calls down fire from the heavens asserts the tradition, which from a sacromagical or theurgic perspective is said to be derived historically from Persia, Assyria, and Babylon.

The esoteric tradition asserts, ultimately, that Middle Eastern temples and religions were the heirs to the lost Fire Temples of Atlantis. While the historical Fire Temple tradition has substantial evidence to support it, the perennial esoteric tradition of Atlantis is found only in some fragments from Plato, who claimed to be quoting an ancient tradition. Most of the widely disseminated "Atlantean" references found today in New Age literature are likely to be fiction. Nevertheless, the tradition is upheld on the inner planes, and is of value to us [35].

The key image and concept is always: Fire over Water. The classic emblems are the pyre that burns when wet, the volcano rising out of the ocean, or the artificial sacred mountain, as in the pyramids of Mexico, South America, and Egypt [2].

The Fire Temple tradition is behind the works of Empedocles (circa 490-430 BCE), the volcanic Sicilian metaphysical philosopher who is credited with the earliest references to the Four Elements, which he termed the Roots of the cosmos, Elements being a term later developed by Plato. There are many interconnected Fire references, as we might expect, in *Aesch Mezareph*.

Elisha is the heir to Elijah in the prophetic fire tradition. He is a "prophet of natural wisdom". This refers not only to manifest nature, but to the supernal Wisdom of the Tree of Life, which can, under certain circumstances flow as a Lightning Flash to ignite substances in nature. There are many other verses and sources on Wisdom with which the original author would have expected the reader to be familiar. The modern reader's lack of familiarity with the traditional source texts is a burden, but we have resources for research now that were unknown in the past. Some academic or textual website addresses are given in our Notes for further study, as physical library access might be daunting for research into many of the sources.

The Supernal Triad Emerges from the Void

The three supernal Emanations are Crown or Spirit, Wisdom, and Understanding. The path between Wisdom and Understanding is Judgment, the deepest level of perfect comprehension. Hence Elisha despises material riches, as the greed for wealth is barren, and such greed isolates the individual from deeper consciousness. According to the allegorical use of the story from the *Book of Kings*, the prophet's refusal of a substantial reward for cleansing Naaman is deeply significant. It advises us that spiritual transformation is not to be bought or sold as a commodity, with the further more subtle message that Elisha refuses reward because of the consciousness that such reward implies or generates.

Later in the original story we discover that the prophet's deceitful servant, *Gehazi*, runs after the Syrians to claim the reward for his self and then hides it. While there is a simple moral teaching in the Old Testament or Hebrew source, the alchemical and spiritual allegory is that greed for material riches leads to a fortress mentality, shutting up the hoarded wealth. As result, the prophet punishes his servant, not for greed in claiming a reward that had already been declined, but for lying about his actions. The *consciousness of an action* is everything in theurgic, sacromagical, and alchemical operations. The name *Gehazi* means "valley of avarice", so this unfortunate servant has become, through his greed and ignorance the materialist antithesis of the Supernal Emanations. The allegory is one of energy and consciousness running and returning (as Gehazi does) in an imbalanced or impure state.

Elisha, in this context, is also a healer, and here we have a classic alchemical allegory in the purification of Naaman, who was a military leader (from Syria, and therefore not Jewish) suffering from leprosy. Naaman is told to bathe seven times in the River Jordan to effect his cure. Unless we follow, or already know, the Biblical verses referenced, we can miss this significant ritual, as it is not directly quoted in the source text. As always, the author assumes that the reader will be familiar with the reference, found at 2 Kings 5: 1-16.

The Sevenfold Immersion

Bathing impure material seven times (as is required of Naaman) is a typical alchemical sequence, and refers to the elevation of a metal through the Seven Planetary Influences...an ascension of the Tree of Life through Moon, Mercury, Venus, Sun, Mars, Jupiter, and Saturn. While it may seem obscure to the modern reader, it was a standard concept in the ancient world so there was no need for our original author to state it openly, as he expects us to either be familiar with or to read the verses that he references, and to know, for ourselves that they have a hidden meaning. He develops several chapters of *Aesch Mezareph* technique all based on exactly this idea, that the materials or metals can be transformed by the Sevenfold Influences, which he describes in detail. Elisha is "naturally rich", as he is able to heal and bring forth prophecy from the deepest levels of spirit, in the ancient Fire Temple lineage. This theme of natural richness appears to be denigrating of materialism, and at its first level, it is just that. But there are hidden implications, and a specific method of working, concealed yet open to the reader.

Ethics, Needs, and Wants

According to what is said in Pirke Aboth, viz., Who is rich? (Answer:) He that rejoices in his portion. For so the true physician of impure metals has no outward show of riches, but is rather like the Tohu of the first Nature, empty and void. Which word (Tohu) is of equal number with the word Elisha, viz., 411. For it is a very true saying in Baba Kama, fol. 71. col. 2. The thing which causes riches, (such as natural wisdom) is supplied instead of riches themselves.

The *Pirkei Avot* or *Ethics of the Fathers* is a compilation of the ethical teachings and maxims of the Rabbis of the Mishnaic period (70-200 CE). *Pirkei Avot* are found in the Mishnaic tractate of *Avot*, the penultimate in the order of *Nezikin* in the *Talmud*. *Pirkei Avot* is the tractate that explores ethical and moral principles without significant recourse to the substantial body of *halakha* or defined laws found in the *Talmud* that are the foundation of Jewish religious life and study. *Baba Kama* is part of the First Gate of the Babylonian Talmud [29], and deals exhaustively with legal matters. While the modern reader might have some difficulty finding the quote given above, the message remains clear: the laws of ethics are essential to a purified consciousness which, in turn, is essential to alchemical transformation.

In the simplest sense we should focus on the words "The thing which causes riches is supplied instead of riches themselves". This means that if you have natural wisdom, you are able to generate whatever you need, providing that you "rejoice in your portion" and understand what your real needs are, and how they are to be provided. Essential "needs" are not always the same as "wants".

The River of Judgment

Learn therefore to purify Naaman, coming from the North, out of Syria, and acknowledge the power of Jordan: Which is as it were Jar-din that is the River of Judgment flowing out of the North.

The Jordan river's name in Hebrew is *Yarden*, from *yarad* to "descend" or "flow down". Here the unknown author offers us a hyper- reference again, possibly to *Amos 5.24: But let Judgment run down as waters, and righteousness (Justice) as a mighty stream.* Both the topography and etymology of the Jordan are employed here as part of the spiritual teaching. The physical river Jordan, sacred in the Middle East from ancient times, flows from North to South or *downwards*. This is intentionally linked to the idea of descending from Above to Below: the sacred river has become the expression of the cosmos, as in other traditions such as that of the Ganges or the Amazon. We will discover shortly how his tradition relates to the Nile, the other sacred river that played a major role in Jewish history.

Further into the multi-leveled imagery we find that Judgment flows down from Above (the Supernal Emanations) to Justice or Righteousness in action in the Solar and Sub-Lunar worlds of the Tree of Life. The original author expects us to know the various references and to understand from his hyper-references that a stellar spiritual power is the true subject of his discourse. Just as the river Jordan purifies Naaman after seven immersions, so will a stellar stream, flowing from Above to Below, purify whatever substance is immersed in its forces seven times.

There is a further traditional implication that imbalanced power or disease, leprosy, as with the emissary from the King of Syria, healed by Elisha, may seem at first to come out of the North, the place of restriction, breaking- down, and transformation. The alchemical reference to leprosy describes the potential corruption of a specific substance. But the River Jordan, or Jar-din, also flows from *North* to *South*. This is the River of Judgment, from the 3rd and 2nd Emanations of Understanding and Wisdom, down from the Stars in the North, especially the Northern Polar Stars, to the Earth in the South, just as the physical Jordan river flows *down* from Syria.

Leprosy was regarded as incurable in the ancient world, but certain forms of the disease could be ritually or formally cleansed or purified. The word *cured* is seldom used, but the words *cleansed* or purified are often found in a Biblical or Kabbalistic context. We should think of the Sevenfold Bath of Naaman as a process of cleansing of impurities, at its basic level, then of elevation or evolution through the planetary spheres and into the Supernal Emanations that are behind the Planets as great spiritual powers. The physical Jordan is a river of water, but the spiritual Jordan is a river of fire, especially of stellar fire. While our source is Jewish, and not Christian, the traditions persisted, of course, into the time of Jesus. The hidden mystery of the Jordan as a river of Purifying Fire is the esoteric meaning of the baptism story related of John the Baptist and Jesus (Matthew 3.11).

The Descending and Ascending Rivers

Later in Aesch Mezareph (A.M. 7), the mystery of Jordan or Jar-din is again referred to : *JARDEN denotes a Mineral Water, useful in the cleansing of Metals, and Leprous Minerals. But this Water flows from two sources, whereof one is called Jeor, i.e., a fluid, having the Nature of the Right Hand, and very Bountiful. The other is called Dan, Rigorous and of a sharp Nature.*

Jeor (Yeor) is the Hebrew term for a river, and specifically used for the river Nile. *Dan* is the Hebrew term for Rigorous Judgment. Thus this second reference to the River of Judgment referred to in A.M.7 is a fusion of Bounty and Rigor, the 4th and 5th Emanations, or Jupiter and Mars. This river, like the Nile, flows from *South* to *North*, from *Below* to *Above*, ascending the Tree of Life through the stages of elevation and transformation. The two Rivers, Descending and Ascending, together comprise the entire Tree of Life. The descending river emanates toward expression, issuing out of the void (*tohu*), into manifestation as nature, ultimately (from our perspective) on planet Earth. The ascending river rises from the center of our planet Earth (or indeed, any planet), radiating an expanding sphere of Earth Light, into the cosmos.

This descent and ascent is modeled through the Dragons of bardic imagery, colored Red and White, as in Alchemy, referred to as the Involutionary and Evolutionary Streams [2]. A.M.7 continues: *But it flows through the Salt Sea, which ought to be observed, and at length is thought to be mixed with the Red Sea; which is a Sulphurous Matter, Masculine, and known to all true Artists.*

Here the author refers to the White and Red seas, which are also found as the Rivers of Blood and Tears in the European faery tradition, and the rivers of fire and ice in classical Greek and Roman tradition [4]. While the manifest examples are the Dead Sea and the Red Sea, these are embodiments of UnderWorld waters, essential to transformation, hence the connections to passing through the UnderWorld at death.

Of considerable interest as a cross-reference is Ezekiel 47: 1-25, which describes a river flowing from the altar of the Temple, and descending in an alignment according to the Four Directions, its depth increasing according to the height of the Zones of the human body (i.e. ascending the Tree of Life), and its correlation to the Salt and Red Seas mentioned above.

The physical Red Sea has been so named in various languages, such as Latin *Mare Rubrum*, or Greek *Erythra Thalassa*, since ancient times. The color of the Red Sea is traditionally associated with the direction South, as ancient attributions of the Directions were typically given colors. There is an implied connection to the red color of Edom, from the red minerals of the mountains that border the Red Sea. We will return to Edom later. A.M.7 continues:

But know thou, that the Name Zachu, i.e., Purity, being multiplied by 8, the Number of Jesod, produces the Number Seder, i.e., Order, which is 264. Which Number is also contained in the word Jarden; thus you may Remember, that at least Eight Orders of Purification are required, before the true Purity follows.

The author of *Aesch Mezareph* knew, of course, that the number of *Yesod,* Foundation, Moon, is not 8, but 9, though this is explained by Westcott in a footnote as follows: "Eight; how is this? Jesod is the Ninth Sephira, yet Jesod is ISUD ; 10, 60, 6, 4, or 80, lesser number 8. Seder, order, SDK, 264 ; which equals 33 ; Zachu multiplied by 8." [21]

This may be why the original author of *Aesch Mezareph* says "at *least* Eight Orders of Purification are required". The number of Purity is 33, which when multiplied by 9 gives 297, which adds to 18, which resolves again to 9, the number of the Foundation, Moon.

Changing Direction

Now we can return to A.M.1:

And remember that which is said in Baba Bathra, fol. 25, col. 2. He that will become wise, let him live in the South; and he that will grow rich, let him turn himself toward the north, etc. [26].

Although in the same place Rabbi Joshua Ben Levi says, let him live always in the south, for whilst be becomes wise, at the same time he becomes rich. "Length of Days is in her right hand, and in her left, Riches and Honour." Prov., c.3, v.16. So thou wilt not desire other riches. (31)

The *Aesch Mezareph* tells us that the flow of energies from the Seven Directions must be understood and worked with, in order to bring transformation. To become wise, live in the South. The South is the lower hemisphere, the manifest world. The North is the upper hemisphere, the Celestial world. To some extent this links to the astrological map with its horizon and upper and lower fields for the Twelve Signs. We may find wisdom by experience in the manifest world, and transformative forces, often difficult, typically come from the North.

The hidden practice here is to affirm the Seven Directions, and to place yourself in the South, while facing North. This must be done in alignment with the planetary Directions, and not in any arbitrary or abstract way. The practical Kabbalist would have been reminded of the practices advised in *Sefer Yetzirah* [14]. Our Sphere of Art practices are a modern version, with a number of new developments, based upon traditional clues.

The Emanations and the Metals are at One

But know that the mysteries of this wisdom differ not from the superior mysteries of the Kabbalah. For such as is the consideration of the predicaments in holiness, the same is also in impurity;

Here the author starts a new phase of the instruction: *natural wisdom*, he advises, does not differ from the *superior mysteries*. The term "predicaments" does not refer to difficult situations, as in its contemporary use, but is used in its older meaning from the formal discipline of Logic. In Logic a *predicament* (related to the word and concept of *predicate*) is a category or class that can be assigned to something. The predicaments in holiness are the classes of Emanation, the *Sephiroth,* of spiritual nature, whilst those in impurity are those in manifest nature. More simply, we can use the originative map of the Tree of Life, Emanations, and Planets, to guide in our actions in the manifest or expressive world of nature. Why? Because natural wisdom, regarded as a spiritual principle (*Chokmah* or Wisdom, the second Emanation of the Tree of Life) pertains to all worlds.

...and the same Sephiroth which are in Atziluth, the same are in Assiah, yea, the same in that kingdom, which is commonly called

the mineral kingdom; although their excellency is always greater upon the spiritual plane.

Here the same statement is repeated, but using Qabalistic terminology. The same *Sephiroth* or Emanations in *Atziluth*, the supernal and originative world, are in *Assiah*, the manifest world or Kingdom. The spiritual forces are in the metals in the earth, though they are less exalted than when in the spiritual realm alone. The message, as with all theurgic or alchemical methods, is that we are going to be told how to exalt them, how to bring them to their natural excellence through natural wisdom.

Therefore the metallic root here possesseth the place of Kether, which hath an occult nature, involved in great obscurity, and from which all metals have their origin; even as the nature of Kether is hidden, and the other Sephiroth flow from thence.

The *metallic root* (here) is the seed of potential from which all metals have their origin. The mystery of that which is in the earth, in the body of the planet (and in the human body), mirrors the obscure nature of *Kether* the hidden Crown of the Tree of Life, the source from which the other Emanations flow. Here we are reminded that the River Jordan flows from Above to Below, and it is the River of Judgment flowing downwards and becoming Justice. What is missing here is the last of the Three Wheels, that of Fortune...but our author will come to this in his obscure Kabbalistic manner, because by following his instructions, we will change our endless circling of the Wheel of Fortune, and rise through Justice and Judgment toward the Crown or *Kether* . This process is shown in Figure Eight (The Three Wheels). By the time the texts reaches chapter 7, the river has begun to ascend, as described above.

Intentional Confusion May Provoke Thought

From this point on we find the typical obfuscation of the order of the Emanations or *Sephiroth* and the metals or substances associated with them. At the close of an intentionally scrambled set of attributes the author says : *But if anyone hath placed those things in another order, I shall not contend with him, inasmuch as all systems tend to the one truth.* Here is a classic clue that there is another order, and we can set it out stage by stage. Dr. Westcott introduces the text as follows:

"The Aesch Mezareph is almost entirely Alchymical in its teachings, and is suggestive rather than explanatory in its words. The allegorical method of teaching runs through it, and the similes have to be kept carefully in mind, otherwise confusion will result. Several Alchymic processes are set out, but not in such a way that they could be carried out by a neophyte; any attempt to do so would discover that something vital was missing at one stage or other" [22].

We may be reminded of a similar confusion from a more popularized magician, associated with Dr. Westcott, that of Aleister Crowley, centuries after *Aesch Mezareph* was written. Crowley claimed to have received his insights on from an inner contact called *Aiwaz*, who taught him, referring to a possible connection between Hebrew letters, tarot trumps, and the paths of the Tree of Life: "All these old letters of my Book are aright; but *tzaddi* is not the Star."

We cannot discuss here the validity of Crowley's source, but the result was the publication of another classic divide-and-confuse strategy, because if the Hebrew letter referred to as *tzaddi* is not The Star, and if all the old letters are correct *except only tzaddi*, then it must be exchanged with another, which would mean that the "all correct" is further disrupted....and so on. *Tzaddi* is the first letter in the word *tzaddik*, or righteous one (saint). I only mention this well- known 20th century example as people are still pondering (and arguing) over it to this day, when in fact Crowley was merely following an old tradition of willful yet meaningful randomization as found in many Qabalistic texts. We might hope that one of the aims of this process is to encourage research and original thinking, rather than slavish adherence to a dogmatically "correct" text.

Correcting the Metals

Returning to our source text: *Lead hath the place of Chokmah, because Chokmah immediately proceeds from Kether, as it immediately comes from the metallic root, and in enigmatic similes, it is called the "father" of the following natures.*

Lead is usually associated with *Binah*, the third Emanation, that of Understanding, of the containing Vessel for the cosmos, the Divine Feminine, the Great Goddess of Time and Space. Here is the first of the series of associations out of place, though not so far out of place as to seem ridiculous, and intentionally described in such a way as to give forth easy clues.

Lead is associated with the Planet Saturn, originally the 7th Planet and "furthest out", as it was thought, in the Solar System. The Tree of Life, however, has two Emanations beyond *Binah*, making up the Supernal Triad of Crown, Wisdom, Understanding (*Kether*, *Chokmah*, and *Binah*).

When the Planets Neptune and Uranus were formally discovered in the 18th century (though they been observed in previous centuries), they took their seats, so to speak, in association with the higher Emanations. The Planets were always there, of course, as were the Supernal Emanations in Qabalistic and Hermetic magic and mysticism. When Pluto was discovered in 1930, modern Qabalists proposed that this "new" planet would relate to the mysterious non-sphere of *Daath* or Knowledge that crosses the Abyss between the Lower and Supernal Emanations.

Despite the well-established traditional association of Lead with *Binah* and Saturn, our author tells us that lead "immediately comes from the metallic root" just as "*Chokmah* immediately proceeds from *Kether*". He is encouraging us to remember that lead within the earth is the lowest or heaviest of the traditional metals, that is converted upwards by ascending the Tree of Life. Thus it proceeds from the metallic root in the Earth "and in enigmatic similes it is called the father of the following natures" i.e. of those metals that follow in the remaining text, but also of the natures or predicaments of the sequence of planetary metals.

From the traditional Qabalistic perspective this is not as confusing as the modern reader might at first think. The Emanations of the Supernal Triad were frequently thought of as mutually partaking of one-another, especially Wisdom 2, and Understanding 3, the polarized spiritual powers that emerge from infinite Being or the Crown 1. By comparison, the lower Triads of the Tree were further polarized on each extreme, but coming together androgynously or harmoniously in the center. This pattern of relationship is shown in Figure Seventeen. Traditionally the second Emanation, Wisdom, was further associated with the Twelve Signs of the Zodiac, while the first, the Crown, was associated with the *Primum Mobile*, shown by a nebula today, or first movement of Stars out of the Void. This Void is the same *tohu* referred to above, the Nothing out of which all Being emerges.

In alchemical variants Salt is often referred to *Chokmah*, Wisdom, Neptune, while Crystal (Sulphur crystals or quartz crystal depending on the branch of Alchemy or the working experiment) is often ascribed to the Crown, *Kether*. Such attributes may vary, or be allegorically concealed in many ways.

So our author, reminding us of the evolution of metals in the Earth from the seed and hidden root of Being, refers Lead to the Supernal Triad issuing from the Crown of the Tree of Life. But by placing Lead in *Chokmah*, Wisdom, rather than *Binah*, he enables his further intentional dupes.

Tin (should be Lead) *possesseth the place of Binah, shewing age, by its greyness, and shadowing forth severity and judicial rigour, by its crackling.*

Here the text should read Lead, which is gray, severe and judicial (Saturnine), though it does not crackle. In A.M. 4, Tin is correctly associated with *Zedek,* the planet Jupiter (Emanation of Mercy, *Chesed*).

The clue is found in the attribution of severity and judicial rigor, which are the next octave downwards from Understanding 3, toward Severity 5, and still associated with certain Saturnine qualities. Here is another hyper-ploy, for Tin is not traditionally associated with *Binah* 3 Understanding, Saturn, but with *Chesed* 4 Mercy, Jupiter, the polar Emanation to *Geburah* 5 Severity, Mars. The corrected metallic association for Mars is Iron, which is described in A.M.3.

Silver (should be Tin) *is placed under the Classis of Chesed, by all the masters of the Kabbalah, chiefly for its colour and use.*

Here our author seems to suddenly run out of steam, for he knows full well that Silver is not placed under the classis of *Chesed* 4 Mercy, Jupiter, by all masters of the Qabalah, and that Silver is associated with *Yesod* 9 Moon, Foundation. But he has given enough clues above to anyone versed in the planetary affiliations and powers.

The White and Red Natures

Thus far the white natures. Now follow the red.

As white and red are of significance in the esoteric traditions, we should consider this cryptic comment carefully. The White Natures are said to be Lead, Tin, and Silver. There are three of them, but Tin and Silver are seemingly misplaced. Does he imply that the White Natures partake of Saturn/Neptune, Jupiter/Mars, and the Moon? This would make a long Triad between the Supernals and the Foundation, and a further long Triad between Jupiter/Mars, being the Emanations of Mercy/Severity and the Foundation or Moon and Sub-Lunar world as shown in Figure Eighteen (The Long Triads). Neither of these Triads is shown on a standard Tree of Life, so their implication should be of special interest in sacromagical work and meditation.

Gold (should be Iron) *is placed under Geburah, according to the most common opinion of the Kabalists; Job in c.37, v.22, also tells us that gold cometh from the north, not only for its colour, but for the sake of its heat and sulphur.*

This is the first of the Red Natures: Iron and Mars, Severity.

The quote from Job is "*Gold shall come from the North from the wonderful majesty of God.*" (or variants thereon according to translation). Remember how the adept of Natural Wisdom, like Elisha, knows to be established in the South, facing North? Location is everything.

Iron is the traditional metal and energy for Mars, *Geburah*, Severity, the 5th Emanation, and that it should be gold, always associated with the Sun, is certainly not "the most common opinion of the Kabalists". Here the author would have been certain that few would be fooled, but that we are being given a clear clue about the correct order...iron for Mars, Gold for the Sun.

Iron (This should be Gold, the traditional metal for the Sun) *is referred to Tiphereth* (Iron is actually referred to Geburah and Mars; Iron and Gold have been exchanged by the writer.)

So this should read; Gold is referred to Tiphareth (the Sun) for he is like a man of war, according to Exod., c.15, v.2, and hath the name of "Seir Anpin", from his swift anger, according to Psalm 2, v.ult., "kiss the son lest he be angry."

Gold is traditionally referred to *Tiphareth*, 6, Beauty, the Sun. The rest of the passage, however, might be thought of as referring to *Geburah*, Severity, and not to the Sun. The reference to *Exodus 15* covers several verses, not only verse 2, referring to mightiness and warrior qualities, likewise the reference to Psalm 2, last verse. Here the author is proposing the Severe Aspect of Gold, or the Purifying Fire of the Sun.

The Solar Emanations, Lesser Countenance, and *Shekinah*

However, the words *Seir Anpin* are something else: for our author is cryptically referring to *Zeir Anpin* or the Lesser Countenance, called *Microprosopus*, as distinct from the Great Countenance or *Macroprosopus*. The Lesser Countenance or Face is the constellation of Emanations around the central 6th Solar Emanation, of *Tiphareth* or Beauty and Harmony. This Solar constellation is sometimes referred as that of the "emotional" *Sephiroth* or Emanations: *Chesed, Geburah, Tiphereth, Netzach, Hod* and *Yesod*.

These are Emanations 4,5,6,7,8, and 9 as shown in Figure Nineteen (the Solar Emanations). So we must untangle the Severity references, which are attributes for Iron and Mars, and distinguish the Beauty reference, which is for the Lesser Face of Divinity, whereby there is a constellation of polarities around Gold and the Sun. One of the mystical tasks associated with the Lesser Face in Qabalah is a re-union with the *Shekinah* or liberating spirit of the Feminine. This requires, according to the secret tradition, a drawing up of the Lunar Triad into the Solar Triad, which it should be observed is both a sexual theurgy and an ascent of the metals.

Netzach and Hod (Copper and Quicksilver) are the two median places of the body, and the seminal receptacles, and refer to the hermaphroditic brass. So also the two pillars of the Temple of Solomon (referring to these two Sephiroth) were made of brass, I Kings, c.7, v.15.

The Biblical quote from 1 Kings' 13-16 is thus:

13: *"King Solomon brought Hiram from Tyre.*

14: *He was a bronze worker, the son of a widow from the tribe of Naphtali; his father had been from Tyre. He was endowed with wisdom, understanding, and knowledge for doing any work in bronze. He came to King Solomon and did all his metal work.*

15: *He fashioned two bronze columns, each eighteen cubits high and twelve cubits in circumference...*

The reference to the Temple of Solomon and the brass or bronze pillars is a classic Qabalistic hyper-reference, for it offers the *Mystery of the Shekinah within the Prepared Temple*. This is the foundation for the esoteric imagery found in the Waite and Colman-Smith tarot trump of The Priestess.

The 7th and 8th Emanations are Venus and Mercury or Victory and Glory, Exaltation and Scintillation. Traditionally they are always associated with Copper for Venus and (of course) Mercury or Quicksilver for Mercury. Yet our author tells us that they are of Brass, and that brass is hermaphroditic. This is a sexual inference, for the *two median places of the body* are the genitals, as are *the seminal receptacles.*

Suddenly our author, at this point ignoring metallic mercury and copper altogether, has skipped from a metallic planetary exposition to a sexual one, couched intentionally and with multiple layers of meaning, within the Temple of Solomon imagery from the Bible.

The story of Hiram, essential to the Masonic tradition and much explored in many books, has a Qabalistic meaning in its Biblical context, for Hiram, a metallurgist who casts the bronze or brass hermaphroditic or alloyed pillars in a furnace, is endowed with Wisdom/*Chokmah,* Understanding/*Binah,* and Knowledge, sometimes translated as "cunning" meaning *skilled*. Not only must we have the secret source of spiritual fire, but we must also have the skill to work with it.

This triad of Wisdom, Understanding, and Knowledge, bringing the Supernal Emanations into a manifest form through knowledge and skill (*Daath* to *Tiphareth*) is mirrored into the lower triad founded on Victory/*Netzach* and Glory/*Hod,* represented by the metals copper and mercury.

The word "brass" freely used at least as late as the 17th century to refer to a number of alloys, was loosely interchanged with "bronze" and is widely known because of its repeated use in the King James Bible. Brass, however, is made from copper and zinc, so the hermaphroditic brass is an alchemical allegory, as neither brass nor bronze are made from copper and mercury (quicksilver).

While there is no proof, we might be tempted to think that some marginal notes or commentary have been interpolated here, as was often the case when hand-written sources were circulated, sometimes for generations, among initiates and students in Kabbalistic groups, and only put into print at much later dates, often by translators. Our anonymous author, after this significant digression (if it is really a digression), returns shortly to the metals Copper and Quicksilver for Venus and Mercury, and brass is expounded in A.M.7.

Venus and Mercury represent the polarities of thought and feeling, and the mixture of male/female in the human consciousness. When they join together, they become the Hermaphrodite...the perfect fusion of Hermes (Mercury) and Aphrodite (Venus). The body zone reference is significant, for it is the hips, loins, and genitals, the Triad of 7th 8th and 9th Emanations, the subtle force of Venus, Mercury, and the Moon.

Uplifting the Lunar Triad

The relationship of Venus Mercury and Moon, clearly shown on a standard Tree of Life, is the Lunar Triad that must, according to the "hidden" tradition, be *uplifted* into the Solar Triad. A method is offered here, a significant clue to one of the major works of spiritual Alchemy.

While much of the text is occupied with what appears to be a metallic alchemical system, this Triadic method is also described at the outset. It should be combined with the idea and practice of the *tohu* or Void, and the outpouring from North (Above) to South (Below). From the Solar Triad, the entire fusion is uplifted into the Stellar or Supernal Triad. This is that other River, of Rigor and Bounty, flowing from South (Below) to North (Above) and returning to its Source, as described in A.M.7.

The Two Faces, or Long Triads of the Solar and Stellar Realms

The long Triads referred to above are expressions of the Greater and Lesser Face (Figure Eighteen) and may be elucidated as follows:

First Long Triad of the Greater Face, downward reaching: 2-3-9, Wisdom, Understanding, Foundation, or Neptune, Saturn, Moon. The substances are Salt-Lead-Silver (described as "white"). The colors are white for Salt, dark for Lead, and white for Silver. Remember that Lead has a native bright white or silver color when scraped free of any surface oxidization. This property of lead renders it both White and Dark, Supernal and Infernal. Note that our author makes a similar leap from a spiritual root of "lead" in the heavens, to a material root of Lead in the Earth, as described above.

First Long Triad of the Lesser Face, downward reaching: 4-5-9, Mercy, Severity, Foundation or Jupiter, Mars, Moon. The metals are Tin/White, Iron/Dark, and Silver/White. Note that each Triad contains two bright or white metals and one dark one; consider their positions on the Tree of Life in meditation.

Second Long Triad of the Greater Face, upward reaching: 7-8-1, Victory, Glory, Crown or Venus, Mercury, Uranus. The substances are copper, mercury, and sulfur or crystal. The colors are red (copper) white (mercury) and red (sulfur). Thus we have two traditionally "red" substances and one white. If we worked with quartz for Uranus, we would have two white and one red. Sulfur, however, can be designated red or white, according to its nature and location within its exaltation or ascent of the Tree of Life, just as Lead can be dark or light.

Second Long Triad of the Lesser Face, upward reaching: 7-8-*Daath*. Victory, Glory, Bridging Knowledge, or Venus, Mercury, Pluto. This triad offers copper, mercury, and (originally) an unknown fusion of the red and white, at *Daath*. As *Daath* is on the Middle Pillar, its potential color would be somewhere in the spectrum of silver-gold-red/clear, as in Moon, Sun, Stars. Thus *Daath* is likely to be the point in an alchemical process at which *Sulfur changes color*, and the Plutonian association of the 20th century reinforces this volcanic UnderWorld power of transformation. There are some powerful meditations if you work with the Triads and then the Hexagrams shown in this triadic pattern of relationship, as in Figure Eighteen.

The Lunar Realm and Living Water

Jesod is argent vive (i.e. Mercury, but should be Silver for the Moon). For to this, the name "living" is characteristically given;

and this living water is in every case the foundation of all Nature and of the metallic art.

The 9th Emanation, *Yesod*, is the Foundation, embodied in the manifest world by our Moon. The traditional metal here is Silver, though we are told it should be *argent vive*, or quicksilver (Mercury). The definition of Mercury as the mysterious "water" of the alchemists is well-known, but metallic mercury belongs, of course, in the 8th Emanation expressed in our Solar System through the planet Mercury.

The Brilliance, Scintillation, and Glory of quicksilver are readily visible in the metal, but these qualities also refer to the planet. To the ancient Greeks it was *Stilbon* a gleaming fast moving light, originally called Apollo in the morning and Hermes in the evening, though by the 4th century BCE the Greeks understood that this was a single rapid bright planet, becoming emblematic of the Messenger of the Gods.

However, we may dive a little further into this Water, having placed Mercury where it truly belongs. Consider: *this living water is in every case the foundation of all Nature and of the metallic art.* We can understand this in a different manner, and the words *foundation of all Nature* is our clue. The Foundation and Moon are associated with all waters, oceans, rivers and tides. Furthermore the Archangel of the 9th Emanation, *Yesod*, is Gabriel, the ruler of the Moon, and all waters. So here we have the living water that is in every case the Foundation of all Nature, and of the metallic art. Gradually we are led into realizing that the Living Water may be Clear, Salt/White, or Sulfurous/Red, according to its source. This polarized water was described in earlier images as the Clear Sea (Galilee) the Salt Sea (Dead Sea) and the Red Sea, through which the River Jordan flows. There are significant transformative meditations and theurgic actions in this sequence.

Coming to Earth

But the true medicine of metals is referred to Malkuth, for many reasons; because it represents the rest of the natures under the metamorphoses of Gold and Silver, right and left, judgment and mercy, concerning which we will speak more largely elsewhere. Here we are reminded that the natural evolution and transformation of metals occurs within the Earth, *Malkuth*. The earthy transformation includes all substances, all metals, subject to the forces of polarity: the metamorphoses of Gold and Silver (Middle Pillar), right and left (Pillars of the Tree of Life) judgment and mercy. And the author does indeed follow up and speak of them again in his subsequent chapters.

Thus I have delivered to thee the key to unlock many secret gates, and have opened the door to the inmost adyta of Nature. But if anyone hath placed those things in another order, I shall not contend with him, inasmuch as all systems tend to the one truth.

We discussed the intentional confusion of the order above, but there are some further hints in these sentences. The "many secret gates" and the "inmost adyta (holy of holies) of Nature" refer to the multiple gates employed in Qabalistic meditation. Fifty Gates are associated with *Binah*, Understanding, the 3rd Emanation, often equated with the relationship between the Ten Emanations and the Five Senses, or the Ten Emanations and the fingers of each hand, totaling 2x5x10, resulting in 100. There are extremely sophisticated methods regarding the many secret gates and the human organs in practical Qabalah [1].

The Three Supernal Emanations as Sulphur, Salt, and Mercury

For it may be said, the three supernals are the three fountains of metallic things. The thick water is Kether, salt is Chokmah, and sulphur is Binah; for known reasons.

The Supernal Emanations are represented here as a Triad, in the process of descent or flowing from Above to Below. As before, Above to Below is the descent of the Tree of Life, North to South, or the flow from the Void toward Manifestation, into expression as the Kingdom/*Malkuth*.

The "three supernals" are, as we might expect by now, intentionally misplaced: Sulphur is *Kether*, Salt is *Chokmah*, and "thick water", a spiritual octave of Mercury (not the metallic Mercury) is *Binah*. This last substance causes much confusion, until we realize that it is alchemical language for *menstruum*. Sulphur is the first fountain, the spirit of stellar fire arising out of the void, as mineral sulphur arises on Earth out of the volcano. Salt is the second fountain, as a multitude of Stars out of the Stellar fire, increasing to infinite numbers just as salt grains are infinite in the ocean of water upon Earth. The Thick Water, within the Vessel of *Binah*, the Great Mother, is the coagulation of the previous forces as they are contained and shaped toward manifestation [30].

A similar allegory of Three Fountains and transmutation from poison to cure is found in the 12th century medieval *Vita Merlini* of Geoffrey of Monmouth, in which a goddess-like figure holds the North in one hand, and the South in the other, after transmuting three fountains of Life, Desire, and Death [3]. Out of the Three Supernals, the modified flow of the River of Judgment pours into the lower Emanations. Once again, the order has been intentionally confused, but is easily rectified. The writer reminds us next of the relationship between the Three Supernals and the Seven Solar Emanations.

The Seven Lower Emanations as the Seven Metals

And so the seven inferior (Emanations) *will represent the seven metals, viz., Gedulah and Geburah, Silver and Gold;* the order is intentionally scrambled, as this refers to the 4th and 5th Emanations, Mercy and Severity (described also as Bounty and Rigor in A.M.7 quoted above). The correct metals are Tin for Mercy/Jupiter, and Iron for Severity/Mars.

Tiphereth, Iron; Netzach and Hod, Tin and Copper; For *Tiphereth*, Beauty/Sun, the 6th Emanation, the correct metal is Gold. For *Netzach* and *Hod*, Victory and Honor, Venus and

Mercury, the 7th and 8th Emanations, the correct metals are Copper and Quicksilver (metallic mercury).

Jesod, Lead; and Malkuth will be the metallic woman, and the Luna of the wise men; and the field into which the seeds of secret minerals ought to be cast, that is the water of Gold, as this name (Mezahab) occurs, Genesis, c.36, v.39.

Jesod, Lead The 9th Emanation is *Yesod*, Foundation, the Moon. The correct metal here is, of course, silver. But what about lead? Lead is associated with Saturn, the 3rd Emanation of *Binah*, Understanding. Here lead is understood as the heaviest metal of the traditional seven, found within the Earth...the force of the 3rd Emanation in metallic form, giving containment and giving weight. So the author, knowing that we shall associated silver correctly with the 9th Emanation, implies that the material octave of Lead must belong to *Malkuth*, which we shall explore shortly. For contemporary people we might meditate on the power of Lead to contain and protect us from radiation. There may also be an implication of an alchemical joke here, for if you scratch lead, it shines like silver, but only the ignorant would be fooled.

Balancing the Kings of Edom

The reference to *Genesis c.36,v.39* refers to the mystery of the *Kings of Edom* that has a convoluted Qabalistic tradition. In the allegorical mode, this is a reminder that all forces must be balanced within the Tree of Life. Traditionally the Kings of Edom are said to represent the peak of force in any Emanation, reigning only until this force is balanced by the next, during the process of creation. Thus Wisdom is balanced by Understanding, Mercy by Severity, and Victory by Honor. Wisdom and Understanding then emit Beauty, and Victory and Honor emit Foundation, and all forces flow into form in the Kingdom, which for us is our manifest world of nature, and planet Earth.

Mezahab means "water of gold", and Mezahab was the maternal ancestor of *Mehitabel*, "rejoicing", the wife of the *last*

King of Edom. This implies that we will rejoice when we are initiated into the mysteries of the true order of the Tree of Life.

Mysteries of the Shekinah and the Ark

Malkuth will be the metallic woman, and the Luna of the wise men; The 10th Emanation is the location for all forces and forms, and is therefore entwined in the Mystery of the Hidden Bride, the *Shekinah* or Divine Feminine power hidden in Nature. As discussed above, the author has exchanged the 10th and 9th Emanations, Lead and Silver. We can simplify all of the above, for *Malkuth* is the starting place, the field in which the seeds are sown for the evolutionary process of ascending the Tree of Life, elevating the Seven Metals through the Tenfold Process.

But know, my Son, that such mysteries are hid in these things as no tongue may be permitted to utter. But I will not offend any more with my tongue, but will keep my mouth with a bridle, Psalm 39, v.2.

As is frequently found with the quotations proposed by our author, we must read more than one verse, and more than one text, to discover the hyper-references here. Psalm 39 has, in its first few verses, more than the caution about silence.

To the chief Musician, to Jeduthun. A Psalm of David.

1 I said, I will take heed to my ways, that I sin not with my tongue: I will keep my mouth with a muzzle, while the wicked is before me.

2 I was dumb with silence, I held my peace from good; and my sorrow was stirred.

3 My heart burned within me; the fire was kindled in my musing: I spoke with my tongue,

4 Make me to know, JHVH, mine end, and the measure of my days, what it is: I shall know how frail I am…

The Psalm is dedicated to Jeduthun "the chief musician". Jeduthun was one of the musicians who "stood before the Ark of the Covenant", and whenever the Ark was moved, was associated with it. Furthermore, the Ark, filled with the Divine power and the radiant *Shekinah* rested for three months in the house of *Obed-Edom* "worshipper of Edom" before being finally located in Jerusalem. Thus the first hint is about the Ark, the Shekinah, and the temporary location in a house of Edom.

The second hint is that the silence builds within until the fire of the heart is kindled. This reminds us of the admonition at beginning of A.M.1 that the truly wise person must be empty and void, as the *tohu*, in order to be filled with the Fire of Purification, and therefore with the potential of prophetic utterance. Thus we have come full circle, and the end is as the beginning. We are now coming to the end of Chapter 1 of Aesch Mezareph.

Gehazi the Servant of Elisha, is the type of the vulgar students of Nature, who contemplate the valley and depths of Nature, but do not penetrate into her secrets. Hence they labour in vain, and remain servants forever. They give counsel about procuring the son of the wise men whose generation exceeds the power of Nature, but they can add nothing to assist in his generation, 2 Kings, c.4, v.14 (for which purpose a man like Elisha is required).

Here the author reminds us that spiritual power is required, not just material information. This spiritual truth is found in another form today in a remarkable premise of quantum mechanics, which proposes that the state of the observer will affect the outcome of any situation or experiment. The esoteric traditions teach that purity of intention, and ethical quality, is essential for any theurgic transformation to occur.

For Nature doth not open her secrets to them, v.26, but contemns them, v.30, and the raising of the dead is impossible to them, v.31. They are covetous, cap. 5, v.20; liars, v.22; deceivers, v.25; prattlers of other men's deeds, 2 Kings, c.8, v.4-5, and instead of riches, contract a leprosy themselves, that is disease, contempt and poverty, v.27. For the word Gehazi, and the word Chol, profane or common, have both the same number.

Dr. Westcott gives an interesting footnote for this passage: "The meaning of this portion appears to be that Gehazi represents the Pretender to Alchymy who knowing that transmutation is possible, wastes his own time, and advises a similar waste on the part of others, in attempting processes against natural law and harmony; one metal cannot be directly turned into another, but the path of evolution must be retraced to the *hyle* or *prima materia* and then the other line of evolution followed." [32]

Conclusion

If you have had the endurance to stay with me for this elucidation, you will have realized just how complex and interactive *Aesch Mezareph* is. A full exposition of all eight chapters would fill a very substantial book indeed, and I am aware that I have barely scraped the surface of Chapter 1 to reveal its hidden depths. What is important for us, as modern people doing sacromagical and theurgic work, is to realize that there is a continuing tradition. The language and the convolutions of the initiates of the past can only be truly understood after spiritual practice, not through analysis without participation. To make gold, you must first have gold.

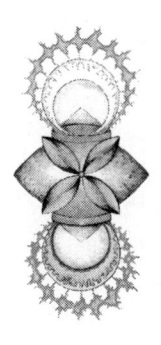

APPENDIX ONE

Preparing and Diluting from a Matrix

As taught in our Fire Temple/*Aesch Mezareph* workshops and classes. The basic method can be applied to your essences prepared according the *Aesch Mezareph* method in our main text, in the section on The Wet Way.

Your Fire Temple Essence will last you for a long time: think of it as being similar to a Flower Essence, but capable of much further dilution. Here are the basic notes for preservation and preparation, followed by some notes on uses for your Fire Temple Essence.

1 The bottle that you filled at the ceremony is your Matrix. Add brandy to it as a preservative. If you wish, you can halve your Matrix into a further dropper bottle, and top up both with brandy. This way it will keep for years. A good proportion is 1/3rd brandy with 2/3rd original. There are no other physical ingredients, and no medicinal contents or claims are made regarding it.

2 Mixing bottle. Your mixing bottle can be the next size up from the matrix bottle(s). Fill this ¾ full with spring water, and add just 3 drops of matrix essence. *Succuss* or pound on your palm thoroughly, at least ten times. You can also add a small amount of brandy from time to time as you use and further dilute the mixture. You can add further spring water, from any clean source, to your mixture when you have used half of it. At this stage you might want to add some further preservative brandy. The mixture can be repeatedly diluted before you need to add any further drops from the matrix solution. The more you dilute it, the more subtly strong it becomes.

3 Storage: keep the matrix and the mixture on or under your meditation altar. If you do not have a permanent altar, keep your essence with a candle that you use for your Sphere of Art work, ideally in a box. Your essence should not be exposed to full or strong sunlight, but does not need to be kept dark.

4 Uses: the mixture contains nothing but water, brandy, and subtle forces. There are no other contents. Thus you can spritz some of the mixture onto your tongue or add a few drops into a glass of water to drink. Try this before a meditation, or when you are fatigued, choosing by Emanation, Planet, or Combination. For general trauma/exhaustion, however, use Five Flower Formula (from Healing Herbs) or, if it is the only one available, Nelson's Bach Rescue Remedy (which is the same formula, but not, in my experience, as resonant).

5 Uses: Make a dilution of the appropriate Essence for spritzing a room, attuning to the Four Directions, Above and Below. Choose it by Planet, Emanation, or Combination. This is very helpful when traveling, and also for subtle cleansing of your bedroom before sleep, last thing at night. You can also spritz some of the essence into a bath, ideally before a ceremony, meditation, or sleep.

6: If you are somewhere that seems unhealthy or inimical, try spritzing to the Four Directions. Always use a compass to find North, and do Not guess or "declare" the Directions. Under really difficult circumstances you can sleep with the appropriate dilution mixture under your pillow or in your hand.

7: Caution: do not give these Essences to anyone. They are attuned to you and your spiritual work. You cannot make them for someone else.

NOTE: Permission is not given to use the methods or resulting preparations described this book to create commercial products.

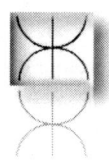

APPENDIX TWO

Working with Inner Contacts

The Nuts and Bolts of Spiritual Communication

This short exploration does not seek to either prove or disprove the validity of spirit beings or communication with the inner planes or metaphysical dimensions. Instead it sets out some guidelines, insights, and conclusions, trusting that readers will discover more for themselves. The overall assumption is that you are aware that there are spiritual dimensions, so time is not wasted in attempting to prove their existence. Only you can prove this to yourself, through a combination of intuition and experience.

There are several levels or modes of spiritual or inner communication, and considerable confusion and misinformation abounds in books and classes on the subject. The basic information, however, has always been available through the centuries, even during the long period of religious suppression. When we examine traditional sources and relevant literature carefully, they all convey similar insights and information, regardless of historical or cultural differences. More serious problems arise when there are politicized religious strictures from powerful vested interests, and all alternative spirituality is condemned, as this significantly suppresses and warps consciousness.

Since the late 19th century, and especially in the latter part of the 20th the huge upsurge of interest in spiritual matters has not been well supported by a commensurate body of research and serious practice; the suppression and confusion inherited by the post-Christian era, combined with the heady sense of liberation (and newly established legal entitlement in some countries), has generated much confusion. False knowledge abounds, as that surging energy of liberation has seldom been applied to study of ancestral wisdom and experience. Hence we find ourselves in situations whereby anyone who has an insight or a presumably spiritual experience in our deprived and materialized world can set themselves up as a leader, teacher, guru, of some sort. Yet such spiritual experiences were once commonplace, and to claim special status one had to prove remarkable spiritual potential and insight beyond that of the widespread visionary and psychic field once shared by the general population, but now seemingly in decline.

It is sometimes asserted that the time of vision and insight has passed, and that consciousness, so crusted with materialism, has declined. This is not so. In truth, everyone, without exception, has spiritual experiences continuously, but they are protectively filtered in general consciousness. In this culture we have many rigid filters, further buffered and enervated by the simulacra of media entertainment, but the unbroken flow of spiritual awareness continues unrecognized, rejected, and frequently medicated in daily life through either prescriptions or so-called recreational substances.

Replacing aggressive punitive religious dogma there is now a huge body of more open and credulous New Age dogma, especially on the commercialized theme of "channeling". This field is long overdue for re-evaluation, as it can, if taken at face value, form a significant barrier to deeper spiritual communication. Rather than single out specific sources of dogmatic misinformation or fantasy for negative criticism, we can consider instead a simple set of guidelines for positively assessing the quality of spiritual communication.

By "spiritual" or "inner" communication we mean the reception and exchange of consciousness between ourselves and beings in metaphysical dimensions. At this stage we are not going to discuss or attempt to define what and where such metaphysical dimensions may be, but merely to affirm their existence. They exist, and there is consciousness within them that can communicate and exchange with us. Nothing more, nothing less. Such communication is seldom in words, but can be brought out, formalized, as words by the recipient if he or she chooses. Expression is always subject to the recipient's skill with words, and there are, of course, many possible areas of confusion in any pre-verbal stage. When we consider that accuracy of reporting in the material world is frequently erratic, and that a group of people will often recount an event or conversation with wildly varying reports, we can begin to understand the problem. As always with such communication problems, a balance must be struck between an outrageously loose subjective response and rigid blinkered literalism that can miss the deeper implications of any interaction.

The basics of spiritual communication, nevertheless, have always been known and taught within the deeper spiritual traditions. In some cases, these basics are described to support dogma *against* spiritual communication and to highlight only "approved" experiences, all others being deemed undesirable. In the perennial subtly hidden traditions the basic knowledge has long been available, and can be further confirmed by repeated experience and common sense. It is this common sense aspect that is most helpful, for communication in the spiritual dimensions will frequently be subject to the same common sense as that of the outer world.

The Basic Information

1: Most spiritual communication is not in words. Only when we begin to understand this will we come more clearly into spiritual communication.

2: It comes instead in formless *intimations* or streams of non-verbal communication. Such intimations may also generate imagery, and this is why ancestral spiritual traditions have collections of images associated with wisdom stories. Prior to the widespread use of written material, religious or sacromagical material, all traditional wisdom, was held in images, either in memory, or in representations such as pictures and carvings. Non-verbal communication is something very familiar to us. Remember that much of our daily interaction and wider consciousness is also non-verbal. The non-verbal of daily life, however, is of a lesser order or slower rate than that of spiritual communication.

3: Typically such spiritual communication will be rapid and condensed. The more advanced or higher consciousness seems, to us, to be instantaneous, and highly concentrated with multiple levels of meaning simultaneously embedded in the content. Thus one rapid sequence of communication may produce, from within us, both words and imagery as we bring it down to the accustomed level of outer form.

4: It is, therefore, the task of the recipient to "translate" or "decode" the communication.

Some Classic Cautions

5: If a spirit contact says "write this down" and starts to dictate detailed word-by-word text this is, undoubtedly, of a low level. Dictated text is, as we may remember, a feature of the human world, and is not relevant within deeper spiritual communication. Once someone has grasped this significant concept, much of the trivia and nonsense around spirit communication can be disposed of, leaving a clearer field. If we consider our own processes of thought and writing, we already have the insights and experience to grasp why dictation, word by word, is never likely to be of much value in spiritual communication.

We always need, and often use, linear speech and text for our outer communication, but we do not *think* in this mode. Consider yourself thinking in a manner whereby you would spell out each word letter by letter in your mind: you never do this. We think relatively swiftly, and the resulting words slow down to express such swiftness, either verbally or, even more slowly, as text. We only need to explore gently our own thought processes to understand why spiritual communication is not rigidly verbal or linearly text based. It exists in dimensions of thought and energy, not solely within the brain or upon the tongue, through the pen, nor by tapping a computer keyboard.

When we consider that spiritual communication is faster than our customary modes of thought, and is more concentrated and intense, we can understand why verbiage based messages from the spirit realm, or even what appear to be friendly neighborly conversations, are so unlikely to be of real value. Unlikely but not uncommon. Most of the textual stuff, dictated teachings and messages, can be judged by its content; is it relevant, what quality does it have? Does it truly reveal spiritual potentials, or is it just verbiage and platitudes? Common sense is a good arbiter.

The faster modes of thought, feeling, cognition, and intuition, are the language of the spiritual dimensions. We know this from our own experience, and with practice can confirm it in meditation. Rather than think of a spiritual language as small units, in words and sentences like our outer language, consider instead that it comprises modes of consciousness that are behind or before outer language. Just as we have the seeds of these modes within ourselves, prior to formal words, so are they the natural communicative means of consciousness, reception and exchange, in metaphysical realms of being.

Communication, therefore, may arise as images, wordless intimations, or abstract symbols; this is why many spiritual or sacromagical traditions have special emblems, icons, or glyphs. Such meta-signs and alphabets are supposed to go beyond the norm, and provide interfaces for communication that can be understood in both the outer and inner dimensions. Unfortunately there is an aura of glamour around the confused fragments of such systems, whereby they are published repeatedly without any real knowledge of their meaning, thus creating yet another backwater in which the traveler can become temporarily lost.

6: The rules of spiritual communication are the same as those of common sense in outer life. If there are mundane "messages" they are of little value. Such messages belong in the trivia of daily life, which is already immensely overloaded. This layer of consciousness, full of mundane messages, may be helpful for those who seek a cautious confirmation of other dimensions, but it is severely limited. We do not naively accept trite "messages" from strangers on the street, or respond with total belief to every telephone solicitation, text message, or email, so why should we accept the equivalent from spiritual sources? The problem of spam messages in email is a helpful comparison, for the psychic dimensions are replete with spam. Just as email is clarified by a spam-filter, we need selective processes and filters for our incoming spiritual communications.

To be clear: I am not denying the validity of spiritual communication, as I am certain that it is very widespread indeed. Most people receive such communication often, but tend to filter it out...just as we filter out most of the input from the everyday world. Such filtering enables us to function in the outer world, but we need a similar filtering in our spiritual exchanges. Fortunately such filters exist, and can also be specially trained into us and created according to our needs.

Some years ago, during the frenzied and often gullible height of the channeling craze, people occasionally wore a T-shirt with the words "Just because they're dead don't mean they're smart". This sarcastic joke carries a significant truth: if your uncle Joe was a loveable but somewhat dull unperceptive person in life, why would his messages suddenly become of cosmic significance after death? Especially as after death there is not much of uncle Joe's personality left, and he moves on to reincarnate anew, perhaps to pursue those wild adventures that were previously closed to him.

On a more serious note, the relatively trivial communications that are often loosely associated with deceased friends or family tend to come from fragmented consciousness at best, or masquerading parasitic consciousness at worst; such contacts work through a feedback pattern, mimicking or broadly suggesting something that the recipient will want to hear in return for a supply of vital energy. In extreme cases this type of communication can build into an unhealthy loop, and create dependence; it should be approached with caution.

7: The faster a spiritual communication is, the more condensed, the less verbal, the more valuable it is likely to be. It is up to us to open-out the communication and judge its value. Contrary to the popular dogma regarding ascended masters many of the condensed packages of communication from other realms of consciousness are noticeably out of touch with the human world. This should not be surprising, for advanced levels of consciousness cannot perceive our world as we do: for this to happen, they would have to limit themselves...in other words, they would have to be us!

Each type of consciousness, personal and transpersonal or meta-personal, is appropriate to function in its own world. Only by *exchanging* can we all know, wherever we are, of the conditions in each dimension of being.

8: The popular idea of Masters (usually *ascended* Masters, and never Mistresses) suggests that there are wise beings that can clearly see and fully understand our world better than we may. This is nonsense, at least in the context of a superior perception. Our understanding is indeed confused, but those advanced or exalted consciousnesses (if we are fortunate enough to contact them) are cut off from our world, by their very nature. They do not have a wise overview of our world, though they do indeed have wisdom on a very different time scale to our own. If a communicating being tells you that he/she/it knows best and you are "not ready yet" you can be sure that it is a fraud or of a relatively low level of consciousness.

When you hear about a plan that is closed to you, you are being given standard dogma that has been around since at least the 19th century, when Theosophy and Madame Blavatsky first popularized the idea of the Hidden Masters and claimed to channel their messages. As somebody once said: "If there are Hidden Masters, what are they hiding from?" Ah...all will be revealed in good time, but you are not ready yet for the greater truth. Meanwhile the Masters will play hide and seek.

Beware of Stereotypes

9: Beware of stereotypes. If a communicating being appears as a stereotype, or tells you that it is some stereotypical person or category of spirit, it is usually a simulacrum or poseur. This is a difficult subject, as there are many soft boundaries and gray zones, but we have to ask ourselves why (for example) the Comte de Saint Germain wastes his immortal time and wisdom dishing out so many thousands of words of platitudes to us through channelers, but seldom come direct to us in our individual meditations with any useful applicable content. The simple answer is that simulacra of *le Comte* abound: they are entities that pose as a stereotype of the popular "ascended master".

This caution regarding stereotypes and simulacra is sometimes unpopular, but is a helpful filter for us. It does not mean that you have to be aggressively cynical, but cautiously practical, slightly skeptical. Astonishing as it may seem, people will embrace the most ridiculous propositions from the "spirit world" which they would never consider in outer life. Common sense is the key: if, by the standards of common sense, it seems somewhat unlikely that your life, or that of someone else, is now being guided by Brahms or Schopenhauer, overlooking blinkered humanity from a higher dimension, then a brief reassessment of such guidance would be healthy. We might add here that a lesson can be found in the quality of the work of those who claim to channel famous composers or philosophers, or any other superficially attractive deceased historic person. Is the channeled material worthy of its supposed or declared source?

10 The spiritual dimensions, which is to say the many modes of non-physical non-manifesting consciousness, teem with beings. Simply expecting communication and opening yourself is like sitting to meditate in the middle of a six-lane freeway, and hoping to encounter only one or two vehicles, and those one or two being of great significance and support and carrying cargo, messages, just for you. Is this likely, or unlikely? Of course there are plenty of beings that want to communicate: often they are the panhandlers and scam-artists of the spirit world. At best they are trying to be helpful, often with resources more limited than your own, *and they mimic what they think you want to hear*. At worst they are parasitic, seeking to trigger your fears, desires, emotions, in order to sustain themselves.

The Neighborhood Analogy

We should take the same common sense action in the spiritual dimensions as we might on visiting a strange city, which is to find a neighborhood that best meets our needs. The neighborhood analogy may be summarized as follows:

a) The streets are generally safe but can be dangerous: (equates to) moving your awareness through the spiritual dimensions.

b) There are bad parts of town where the innocent may suffer: (equates to) straying into areas of psychic imbalance occupied by unhealthy beings that prey upon desires, fears, and addictions.

c) There are welcoming hotels, but you must pay a price, and you can only stay if you pay: (equates to) religious dogmatic sanctuaries in the spiritual world. Open for believers only, closed to all others.

d) There are many other neighborhoods, but we should always explore with caution, respect, and integrity. Equates to daily life!

11: Attunement is everything. What you attune to is ultimately what you get, both in this outer life and in the after-death consciousness. Like attracts like, so if we want good quality spiritual communication, we have to work to clarify both our reception and our transmission. While the analogy is to mechanistic or broadcast processes, our exchange is not, of course, through a machine, but through our living consciousness, our thoughts and emotions, and especially through our imagination.

If the imagination is clouded or overloaded with unhealthy images from media entertainment, clear spiritual communication is most unlikely. A healthy reception and transmission from and to the spiritual dimensions is founded upon a clarified and purified imagination, not upon fantasy or self-indulgent whimsy. None of the above implies that we "merely imagine" spiritual communication; there is no such thing as *mere imagination*, as even self-indulgent fantasy or escapist immature imagery can carry enormous energy, often to the point of self-damage.

12: Most of the above has been about what effective beneficial spiritual communication is Not. So to conclude this short exploration, I will offer some thoughts on what it Is.

The Positive and Beneficial Aspects

a) Beneficial spiritual communication is Inspiring. It breathes new life into us and uplifts us. The higher modes of consciousness are catalysts for our inner energies, exalting them to a renewed vigor.

b) Deeper spiritual communion, coming from advanced consciousness in metaphysical dimensions, is initiatory. This simply means that it kick-starts our inner transformation, and opens the way to new understanding.

c) Unconditional love and compassion are at the foundation of genuine spiritual communication. Not in the sense of a personal love or relationship, for those are the dynamics of life in the outer world of nature, but as a flowing stream from the inner planes or inner worlds, toward our outer manifest world.

d) There can also be a rigor in the energies of spiritual communication; we are not given congratulations, indulgence, or leeway, but are instead brought face to face with our faults, as in a mirror. In this sense, the subtle energies of advanced spiritual communication are transformative, for if we choose to go deeper than the popular surface level of spirit-communication, we must be able to live and to function at such depths. To do this, we have to change.

All Things Reversed

As with all aspects of life in the manifest world of nature, we think we are heading forward, but really do everything, unknowing, in reverse. Despite all of the above discussion and potential elucidation, there is one main effective way of coming into deeper spiritual consciousness, and that is through practice. Not practice at communicating, but ongoing spiritual disciplines such as meditation, theurgic ceremony, or other transformative spiritual arts and sciences. Only by changing ourselves within can we come fully into the consciousness whereby those who have already changed can dialogue with us.

In the interim, we must work diligently to reach half-way in our spiritual practices, and other evolved beings will come to the threshold of our awareness, reaching through the other half of the distance between us. We do this not by crying out for help or advice, but by attuning to the primary spiritual qualities of Life, Light, Love, and Law, Above, Below, and Within, and being Still therein. Within this primary sphere, all other practices are enhanced, and clear exchange is possible.

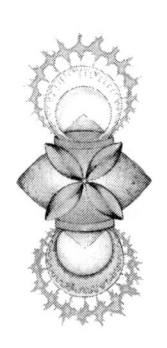

APPENDIX THREE

**THE SPHERE OF ART : Original Audio script, 2009,
From the audio CD "The Sphere of Art"**

The Sphere of Art is a new approach to sacromagical work, based on enduring foundations within the Western esoteric tradition. The method is simple, but it has significant effects on consciousness and energy. There are two main components to the Sphere of Art. The first is the Sphere itself.

The second is the Sanctuary of Avalon as maintained by Ronald Heaver and Polly Wood, with associated esotericists, from the 1950's to 1980. The Sanctuary is now maintained by myself, Robert Stewart with my partner Anastacia Nutt, and our groups in Britain and the USA. The new Sanctuary of Avalon is in a small building on Glastonbury Tor, with further sanctuaries on the east and west coasts of the United States. These manifest sanctuaries lead to the inner or spiritual sanctuary from which the Sphere of Art practices emerge. There are many further esoteric connections to a powerful inner-plane order of Priestesses and Priests, especially associated with the traditional concept of the Fire Temple, with its historical foundations in the ancestral past, and its timeless present in a transformed and uplifted world. When you build the Sphere of Art and attune to the Sanctuary, you can come into your true potential, and discover your spiritual reality that exists beyond time. In this inspirational and training audio, we will focus first on building the Sphere, then on entering the spiritual Sanctuary. The third part is a Tree of Life practice that can be done within the empowered Sphere of Art.

Building the Sphere of Art

To build the Sphere of Art, you should understand that the flat circle so commonly used in magical arts is only the horizontal plane of a sphere. In the big picture sense, the horizontal plane is the surface of the planet on which we stand. In our focused sacromagical work it is a small circle intentionally limited in size to focus spiritual energy. It can be as large as a circle of people, or as small as a sphere around your own body. The Sphere of Art extends upwards to the sky and downwards into the earth. Its height and depth are determined by its circumference...this is the geometric property of all spheres, of course.

The Sphere is built by affirming the classic Seven Directions of Magical Arts: Before you, Behind you, Right of you, Left of you, Above, Below, and Within. These are traditionally defined as East, before you (when you face the rising Sun), West, behind you, South, right of you, North, left of you. You can work facing any of the Four Directions as your starting point, but traditionally East is faced due to the rising Sun and the energy of Beginning that expands and rotates around the Directions.

The upper hemisphere, Above you, has a Sensitive point that admits stellar light.

The lower hemisphere, Below you, has a Sensitive point that admits telluric light, the Earth Light that radiates from the heart of our planet.

The Sphere is established by gentle repetition, rather than forced willpower. It is a microcosm of the planetary, Solar, and stellar forces that create our cosmos.

Building the Sphere.

1: Affirm the Seven Directions. Use the vowel chant, E I O A U. When affirming, let your awareness extend to the limits that you have set for the sphere, before you, behind you, right of you, left of you, above, below, and within the center of the sphere. Do not make the sphere too large...it should be large enough to be harmonious with the room that you work in, or as small as at arm's length all around your body. A group of people defines the sphere by size of the circle that their assembly can make comfortably while standing relatively close together.

2: Acknowledge the Sensitive Points in the uppermost and lowermost parts of the Sphere. The point Below will ideally be somewhat underground. If you are in a multi-storey building, limit the sphere so that it does not intrude into adjoining rooms or apartments. Conceive of above as linked direct to the Stars, and below as linked directly to the earth. Let the structural *substance* of the building work for you, rather than the assorted *contents*.

3: Make your Sphere still, stilling time space and movement. Use the Stillness Chant. OAI.

4: Invoke the Four Guardian Archangels. In the East: Raphael and the powers of Life. In the South: Michael and the powers of Light. In the West: Gabriel and the powers of Love. In the North: Auriel and the powers of cosmic Law.

5: Commune with the Archangels: sense see and feel them as embracing and further defining the shape of the entire sphere. Each Archangel has three pairs of wings. The uppermost pair curves upwards to above, the lowermost pair curves downwards to below. The middle pair extends around the perimeter of the sphere. Sense, see. and feel that the upper wingtips of all four Archangels touch around the iris of the sensitive point Above. Sense, see, and feel that their lower wingtips touch around the iris of the sensitive point Below. The tips of the encircling wings touch at the cross-quarters of the Four Directions.

6: Invite the Archangels to seal the sphere. If you are standing or sitting within one of the Directions, feel the Archangel behind you draw close and touch your spine. In group work each group member mediates this touch to the spine according to his or her location in the Four Directions. If you are sitting or standing in the center, sense, see, and feel all four Archangels at the perimeter of the Directions, but invite the Archangel behind you to touch your spine.

7: Make your Sphere still, stilling time space and movement. Use the Stillness Chant. OAI.

8 Direct your awareness downwards into the radiant Earth Light: let it ascend as a narrow beam through the sensitive point below.

9: Direct your awareness upwards to the Stars: let their stellar light descend as a narrow beam through the sensitive point above.

10: Make your Sphere still, stilling time space and movement. Use the Stillness Chant. OAI. Sense, see, and feel the fusion between the stellar forces and the telluric forces. This fusion forms a New Sun in the center of the Sphere. Contemplate, and commune with the New Sun in Silence.

11: Affirm again the Seven Directions with the Vowel Chant, E I O A U. Invite the Archangels to open out the Sphere. Allow the subtle forces to flow out unconditionally to the Four Directions.

12: Gently extinguish any candles, and return to your outer awareness, using the Crossing Form around your body. "In the name of the Star Father, the Earth Mother, the True Taker, the Great Giver: One Being of Light" AMEN.

The Sanctuary of Avalon Vision

This visionary working should be done within the activated Sphere of Art. You should work with the basic Sphere practice first, and become familiar with it, before you undertake this visionary working.

1: Sense, see, and feel an apple orchard with trees in blossom. It is in a walled garden, behind a large Georgian house. In the garden is a small building standing within the apple trees. This is the Sanctuary of Avalon in Somerset, as it was in from the 1950's to 1980.

2: Pass into the orchard, and approach the building. The wooden door opens, and inside you see a plain and almost empty space, painted white, with a simple altar at the eastern end. A candle burns upon the altar, and there are some chairs and cushions around the room. You pass within, and approach the flame upon the altar. As you do so you become aware of a priestly figure standing behind the altar: this image changes...sometimes it is an elderly man with two walking canes, then it becomes the Priest King of Spirits, a radiant being holding two staffs. Commune a while in Silence with the Flame and the Priest.

Note: This image can be found in the Dreampower trumps, online at www.dreampower.com

3: The wall of the Sanctuary fades to reveal the interior of a mysterious Abbey. The priest leads you into this greater Sanctuary. This is the deep timeless archetype that manifested as Glastonbury Abbey in the historic past. You see the Double Dragon arches in the center, at the Crossing of the Abbey, and you are drawn toward them.

4: Find yourself at the center of the Directions, with the Double Dragon arches before you, behind you, right of you, and left of you. Above are the whirling Stars, below the Earth Light of the regenerative UnderWorld. Be still: commune in Silence. Make the Stillness Chant. OAI.

5: Slowly the Mysterious Abbey fades, and you find yourself back in the Sanctuary of Avalon. Now you are aware of others there with you; they come and go, sitting or standing in silence. Some you may recognize, others are unknown to you. You sense that it is time to leave, and you make a clear commitment to return in your dreams, meditations and waking consciousness. Give thanks and acknowledgement to the guardian priest and those that have gone before us to open the way for us.

6 : You come out into the garden, and discover that you are on the side of Glastonbury Tor, in a small garden of trees, blossoms, and flowers. The Sanctuary behind has changed shape, and become a different building. This is the new sanctuary for the 21st century.

7: Let the image fade, and become aware again of the Seven Directions of the Sphere of Art. Invite the Archangels to release the Sphere. Make the Stillness Chant OAI. Return to your outer awareness.

Note: A further audio meditation and vision of the Mysterious Abbey is included on the audio and music CD of *Advanced Magical Arts*.

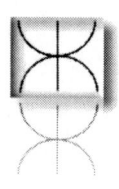

APPENDIX FOUR

Expanding Sequence of Angels

As a general rule definitions in this book have been kept in English, not only as basic translations of any Hebrew words, but in some examples as meditational clarifications of concepts. An expanded glossary of typical Anglicized Hebrew words and concepts used throughout our text reveals many insights into the Tree of Life and the practice of *Aesch Mezareph.*

Emanation, capitalized, is used as an alternative to the typically published words *Sphere* or, in Hebrew, *Sephiroth*, to avoid confusion with other uses of *sphere* or *Sphere of Art* in the main text. **Emanation** has a long tradition as a Qabalistic term, and is a powerful meditational concept when working with the Tree of Life.

The Flow and Return of the Emanations

Emanation is perhaps the best philosophical or metaphysical English word for the powers of the *Sephiroth* or Spheres of the Tree of Life. It helps the meditator to conceive of the powers as successive movements toward manifestation that flow through one-another, rather than as the rigid and artificially visually separated "spheres " and "paths" as shown on a typical Tree of Life map. We can meditate upon the *Emanations* as a set of nested spheres; this is how cosmic maps were drawn in the past, as in our Figure Twenty (The Nested Spheres). The practice has more or less vanished from modern publication.

Figure 20.1 shows the "downward" or Outward Emanations, whereby the successive forces of the cosmos manifest as form . The nested spheres are the Emanations, flowing through one another. This is one of the "hidden" glyphs that generate the standard published Tree of Life.

Figure 20.2 shows the "upward" or Inward Emanations, whereby the successive forces of the cosmos enfold form. This figure reveals the classic Qabalistic mystery of the Crown being present within the Kingdom.

A helpful meditation is to first draw, then to envision without a physical drawing, the two Movements of the Emanations, (Figures 20.1 and 20.2) merged together. This simple diagram reveals connections between the Emanations. For example, 3/2 merges within 7/8, but 4/5 is identical in both sets, while 0/1 merges with 10. Emanation 6 remains constant in both sets, while Emanation 9 merges with 1/2/3. The mystery of the *Shekinah* is hidden in this meditation, along with many other insights.

The Reconciliation of the Worlds

The four fields, clearly visible as the "spaces" *inside* the five nested spheres, may be understood as Origination, Creation, Formation, and Expression, often called the Four Worlds, and widely used in the terminology of Jewish Kabbalah. This Four Worlds concept can be integrated with the Three Worlds of the physical and metaphysical cosmos, which are the Stellar, Solar, and Lunar, enfolding the Ten Emanations. The Stellar World links the fields of Origination and Creation, the Solar World (our Solar System) links the fields of Creation and Formation (for us), and the Lunar World (our Earth-Moon interaction) links the fields of Formation and Expression (here on Earth). Thus do the Five Rings or enfolding macro-Spheres, and their related energetic spaces of the Four Worlds or Fields, reconcile harmoniously with the traditional (and observed) Three Worlds of cosmic manifestation: Lunar, Solar, and Stellar. (See Figures Twenty Eight and Thirty)

The Emanations of the Tree of Life

1 Crown: *Kether,* First Emanation, Breath, Spirit, Being, Primum Mobile, (Uranus/Crystal).

2 Wisdom: *Chokmah,* Zodiac, Star Father, (Neptune/Salt).

3 Understanding: *Binah*, Great Mother (Saturn/Lead).

(No number) Bridging and Knowing {*Daath*, or Knowledge through Experience}

4 Mercy: *Chesed,* Giving, Expansion, Compassion (Jupiter/Tin).

5 Severity: *Jivurah,* Reducing, Purifying, Rigor (Mars/Iron).

6 Beauty: *Tiphareth*, Harmony, Balance, Centrality, (Sun/Gold).

7 Victory: *Netzach*, Power, Exaltation, Ecstasy, Emotional movement, (Venus/Copper).

8 Glory: *Hod*, Honor, Scintillation or Brilliance, Mental swiftness, (Mercury/Quicksilver).

9 Foundation: *Yesod*, (Moon/Silver).

10 Kingdom: *Malkuth*, the Tenth Emanation, Manifest Cosmos, the manifest World of Nature, therefore our Planet Earth. (Earth/Carbon/Volcanic Ash/ All metals, All Substances).

Orders of Archangels and their Angels

The movement of angels toward manifestation (expression) is traditionally expressed and understood in terms of directions, wheels, vessels, or spheres. *All angels are defined by the nature of their movement and the subsequent shape created by such movement.* Thus there is a connection between the *movement* of the orders of angels, the *hewing* or shaping process of *Sefir Yetzirah*, and the expansion and movement of the Emanations in the process described in *Aesch Mezareph*. This sequence, of angelic movement and shapes, offers many insights and possibilities for work within the Sphere of Art. We can describe this movement and shaping as follows:

1 Holy Living Creatures: *Chioth ha Kadesh*, Archangel *Metatron*. [*the primary fourfold voice or breath of Being, coming into Life Light Love and Law throughout the cosmos*].

2 Whirling Wheels: *Ophanim* Archangel *Ratziel* .

[the Holy Living Creatures *move* and this movement generates, and becomes, the Whirling Wheels, *Ophanim*. The *Primum Mobile* and physical nebulae issuing out of the Void, are the manifest forms of this angelic whirling movement, with a further connection to our relativistic Zodiac, Milky Way, and Galaxy, associated with the 2nd Emanation of the Tree of Life, Wisdom, the Star Father].

3 Vessels: *Aralim* Archangel *Tzaphkiel*.

[the Vessels, or more precisely the *rims and curved surfaces* of Vessels or containing spheres, the walls of the vessels rather than the interior space thereof. These angels are traditionally also known as Thrones, the throne being the vessel or seat of power that upholds, contains, and supports the ruler. While a physical throne is a supportive seat, the inherent spiritual nature of the throne is that which contains and enables power in action. Thus the *whirling* action of the *Ophanim* is enclosed or contained, this being the proper power of the 3rd Emanation, *Binah*, Understanding, the Great Mother. Only when energy is contained, force within form, does it act as an engine for further stages of generation.

This enthroning or containing is the cosmic creation process that is studied by our physicists as interactions of energy within space and time. It is mirrored in the containment or interactive union of the energies and orbits of the Solar System, the dynamic pattern of relationship between the Sun and Planets. A further mirroring is the field or sphere that the physical Moon weaves around the Earth, for within this woven sphere, all life on Earth occurs].

Within the originative interactions of the Three Supernal Emanations, the angelic forces are, therefore, cosmological forces, deeply involved in the shaping of space, time, and movement.

Crossing the Bridge

At this point we encounter the Bridge of Knowledge *Daath*, which typically has no traditional angelic or Archangelic beings associated with it, though it is crossed and encompassed by the great Archangelic consciousness of *Metatron*. This *knowledge*, which is not intellectual or factual knowledge, but the deep knowing that comes from experience, bridges the Abyss of Time and Space between the Supernal Emanations and the Planetary Emanations of our Solar System. We can think of it, in manifestation, as the vast space and time that would have to be traversed between our Solar System, galaxy, and the greater cosmos. Descending or coming into expression and manifestation, the Bridge of Knowledge/Experience, *Daath*, is part of the reflective process of the divine Being, whereby the supernal cosmos is mirrored into the manifest cosmos, often traditionally described as an act of *self-knowledge* of the Divine Being. When ascending from expression toward Spirit, the human consciousness or soul crosses the Abyss after death, and can take only what it knows, the essence of what it has experienced, toward a deeper Understanding and Wisdom, as Nothing else is of true value.

Toward the Sacred Earth

4 Generous Brilliant Ones (Radiating, as in a radiant smile), *Chasmalim*, Archangel *Tzadkiel* .

[at this stage the contained vessels from 1-2-3 above are filled to the brim, hence the association of the 4th Emanation, Mercy, with compassion, overflowing, and giving forth].

5 Rigorous Ones, *Seraphim,* (fiery serpents) Archangel *Khamiel*.

[*Seraphim* purify restrict and cleanse with fire. Thus they are the polar partners to the *Chasmalim*. Again, *direction* is significant: "descending" or moving outwards toward manifestation, the rigor of these angels of the 5th Emanation restricts and shapes the ceaseless outflow of the 4th Emanation and causes its generous *forces* to come into balance through the 6th Emanation of Harmony. However, ascending the Tree, the *Seraphim* break down *forms* while cleansing within us the accumulated imbalances of the previous emanations, 9-8-7, associated with the imaginative impulses and the sexual and generative forces. Thus the movement "downwards" mirrors the pattern of wheels and vessels in the Supernal realms, while the movement "upwards" liberates the individual soul toward deeper Understanding and Wisdom].

6 Connecting Ones, *Malakhim,* Messengers, (Spokes of Wheel), Archangel *Michael*.

[Just as angels of the 4th emanation have their outpouring forces shaped and limited by those of the 5th, so does the new Vessel come into Harmony and Balance in the 6th Emanation of the cosmos. The analogy of wheels now becomes associated with the wheel of our Solar System and Planets. The *Malakhim* are angels of the Rod or Spoke, connecting the hub and center, the Sun, to the rim or circumference, the orbiting Planets. *Malakhim* are Messengers because they connect the core or center with the outermost rim, carrying the consciousness and energy to-and-fro, but also strengthening and supporting the wheel in its movement. This Solar wheel is also the Wheel of Justice (shown by the tarot trump of Justice), or perfect poise between Severity and Mercy. Thus the mirroring process completes, with the Second Triad (4-5-6) inversely mirroring the shape and order First Triad (1-2-3).

We can meditate upon the nature of the *Malakhim* in relationship to the *Chioth ha Kadesh*, Holy Living Creatures, for the primary Four that Move have now become the six-fold spokes of the Wheel, and the Declaratory highest angels have now become the Solar Messengers. This relationship is shown in Figure Twenty-One].

7 Life Enablers, *Elohim*, Energizers, Uplifters, Archangel *Auriel*.

[*Elohim* is one of the most frequently discussed words through the centuries of Judaism, Christianity, and, of course Qabalistic mysticism and magic. The word can be, bafflingly for some, both singular and plural, according to context. It is typically translated from the plural as "god-like ones", and this is the angelic context that we refer to here, rather than the singular use of *Elohim* as a divine Name. The *Elohim* (plural) are the angels that Enable Life, or energize potential *lives*, on the way toward expression in Nature, before Life is given its biological Foundation by the *Aishim* and subsequently brought into full manifestation in physical form by the *Kerubim*].

8 Life Activators, *Beni Elohim*, Communicators, Motivators, Archangel *Raphiel*.

[the term *Beni Elohim* can mean "sons of gods/god-like ones" or the *tribe* of the god-like ones. Once again it is used in the plural for angels, as they are always a collective entity. These Communicators, Motivators, and Activators stimulate Life toward both a collective and individual consciousness, on the way toward expression in Nature, after it has been energized by the *Elohim*, and before it is given its Foundation by the *Aishim* and subsequently brought into form by the *Kerubim*. Thus the "higher" orders of angels have their "lower" octaves, which are nevertheless god or goddess-like, and these lower orders are concerned with the manifestation of life and consciousness in the Kingdom, and with the movement into and out of the Kingdom in the cycles of birth, death, and rebirth, for all things].

9 Shining Ones, *Aishim*, Life Guardians, lesser Messengers, Archangel *Gabriel*.

[The *Aishim* are associated with either *Yesod* the Foundation (Moon) or, in some presentations of tradition, to *Malkuth*, the Kingdom. The word is often translated as Souls of Fire, or the souls of holy ones. In effect, the 9th and 10th Emanations are tightly interwoven, and the Foundation was originally understood to be both Earth and Moon as an entity, while the Kingdom was originally understood as the greater manifest cosmos. As the physical Earth and Moon are, in fact, one entity, each revolving around a central point within the mantle of the Earth, this older interaction between the two Emanations is of considerable value to us in meditation.

In our present context, however, we think of the *Aishim* as the Lunar angels of the Foundation. They are the "guardian angels" described in Jewish, Christian, and Islamic tradition. In this sense, if we move beyond cultural religions, they are those spiritual beings that operate in the Lunar and sub-Lunar realms, under the aegis of the greater consciousness that is now called the Archangel Gabriel. Thus these gentle luminous flames bring all beings into birth, and carry them forth again at death. They are the lesser Messengers as a harmonic of the *Malakhim*, just as the light of the Moon is a reflection of the light of the Sun].

10 Elemental Forces: *Kerubim,* Archangel *Sandalphon*, Fourfold Powers in the manifest cosmos, therefore on Planet Earth.

Represented as Eagle, Lion, Human, and Ox and as combination of all four in one: body of Lion, hooves of Ox, wings of Eagle, face of Human.

[the *Kerubim* are the manifest expressed octave of the Holy Living Creatures. Thus they are power-in-motion, the Four Elements in action in the world of Nature. The earliest images are the powerful Assyrian carvings of beings as described above, with composite form. It is likely that this is form taken by the *Kerubim* associated with the Ark of the Covenant, and the *Shekinah* or luminous feminine Presence hovers above and between the *Kerubim*, the radiant divine Being in Her Lunar manifestation].

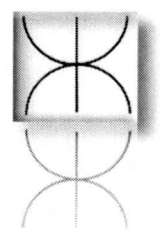

APPENDIX FIVE

The Paths, Tarot Trumps, and the Metals

See also the Tree of Life figures in our main text. The Trumps are illustrated by Merlin Tarot trumps, alternatively by the trumps of the Waite/Colman-Smith deck.

10-9: Sulphur/Carbon and Silver. *Trump of Moon*. Kingdom and Foundation, Earth and Moon.

10-8: Sulphur/Carbon and Mercury. *Trump of Fool*. Kingdom and Glory (Honor, Scintillation), Earth and Mercury.

10-7: Sulphur/Carbon and Copper. *Trump of World*. Kingdom and Power (Victory, Exaltation), Earth and Venus.

9-6: Silver and Gold. *Trump of Sun*. Foundation and Beauty (Harmony, Balance). Moon and Sun.

9-8: Silver and Mercury. *Trump of Magician*. Foundation and Brilliance (Glory, Honor, Scintillation). Moon and Mercury.

9-7: Silver and Copper. *Trump of Priestess*. Foundation and Victory (Exaltation). Moon and Venus.

8-7: Mercury and Copper. *Trump of Fortune*. Glory and Victory. Mercury and Venus.

8-6: Mercury and Gold. *Trump of Chariot*. Glory and Beauty. Mercury and Sun.

8-5: Mercury and Iron. *Trump of Guardian* (Devil). Glory and Severity. Mercury and Mars.

7-6: Copper and Gold. *Trump of Lovers*. Victory and Beauty. Venus and Sun.

7-4: Copper and Tin. *Trump of Empress*. Victory and Mercy. Venus and Jupiter.

6-1: Gold and Sulphur (Crystal). *Trump of Star*. Beauty and Crown. Sun and Uranus.

6-5: Gold and Iron. *Trump of Tower*. Beauty and Severity. Sun and Mars.

6-4: Gold and Tin. *Trump of Strength*. Beauty and Mercy. Sun

6-3: Gold and Lead. *Trump of Hanged Man*. Beauty and Understanding. Sun and Saturn.

6-2: Gold and Salt: *Trump of Temperance*. Beauty and Wisdom. Sun and Neptune.

5-4: Iron and Tin. *Trump of Justice*. Severity and Mercy. Mars and Jupiter.

5-3: Iron and Lead. *Trump of Death*. Severity and Understanding. Mars and Saturn.

4-2: Tin and Salt: *Trump of Emperor*. Mercy and Wisdom. Jupiter and Neptune.

3-1: Lead and Sulphur (Crystal). *Trump of Hermit*. Understanding and Crown. Saturn and Uranus.

3-2: Lead and Salt. *Trump of Judgment*. Understanding and Wisdom. Saturn and Neptune.

2-1: Salt and Sulphur (Crystal). *Trump of Innocent* (Hierophant). Wisdom and Crown. Neptune and Uranus.

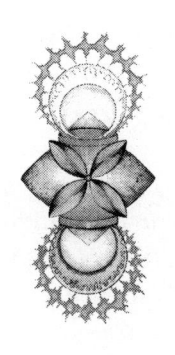

APPENDIX SIX

Preface to the 19th century edition by Dr. Wynn W Westcott. (original spelling has been kept throughout)

The *Aesch Mezareph* or *Ash Metzareph,* is only known to persons of Western Culture from the Latin Translation found in a fragmentary condition in the work entitled *Kabalah Denudata* by Knorr von Rosenroth, published at Sulzbach in 1677-84. These volumes have as a sub-title "The Transcendental, Metaphysical and Theological Doctrines of the Hebrews", and they enshrine a Latin translation, with part of the Hebrew text and commentaries, of the great *Sohar* or *Zohar*, "The Book of Splendour" which is the most famous of all the Hebrew mystical codices of the Kabalah.

The *Aesch Metzareph* is still extant as a separate treatise in what is called the Hebrew language, but which is more properly Aramaic Chaldee: it was a companion volume to the *Chaldean Book of Numbers* so often referred to by H. P. Blavatsky, and which is no longer to be procured, although I have reason to think that copies still exist in concealment. The first volume of Rosenroth's work consists entirely of a Kabalistic Lexicon. Upon the title page is inscribed: *Apparatus in Librum Sohar nempe Loci communes Kabalistici secundum ordinem Alphabeticum concinnati, qui Lexici instar esse possunt.*

Upon the main title page of the work he describes this portion as collected from five sources: *I. Clavis ad Kabalam antiquam: i. e. explicatio et ad debitas Classes Sephiristicas facta distributio omnium nominum et cognominum Divinorum e Libro Pardes. II. Liber Schaare Orah seu Portae Lucis. III, Kabala recentior. Rabbi Jizchak Loria. IV. Index plurimarum materiarum Cabalisticarum in ipso Libro Sohar propositarum. V. Compendium Libri Cabalistico-Chymici, Aesch Metzareph dicti, de Lapide Philosophico.*

The *Aesch Metzareph* can be re-constructed from its fragments scattered through this Lexicon, almost in its entirety. This work has been done by the *Lover of Philalethes,* who published the English version of 1714. The present volume is a reprint of that English version, in its original form; many corrections however, have been made, and a few changes in spelling and diction introduced in order to avoid archaic forms, leading young students into difficulties. For instance, Kabalah is written instead of Kabbala, because the Hebrew word has only one B, and ah represents the Hebrew letter He better than the English a, which suggest that the word is spelled with the Hebrew Aleph.

The Hebrew or Chaldee name of this treatise is spelled thus AShH MTzRP. *The Lover of Philalethes* of 1774 spelled this in English by a diphthong AESCH; and in the second word he puts Z for Tz, Zain for Tzaddi, this leads to confusion and error. The meaning of *Ash* or *Ashah* is "fire" or "a fire offering", and metzareph is "cleansing" or "purifying". The whole title refers to "Cleansing Fires", as the mode by which pure gold was obtained in Alchymy, by burning off the gross and so separating the pure from the impure on the material plane! While the cleansing fire of trial is also a suitable simile for the purification and exaltation of the human soul on the plane of spiritual Alchymy. The words *Ash Metzareph*, or *Aesch Mezareph* as Rosenroth spells it, are found in the book of Malachi, cap. 3, v. 2, where it is said that the messenger of the Lord is like a "refiner's fire". There are in the book many references to other old Hebrew and Chaldee works, several of these are included in the great collection of tracts called the Talmud; of this work there are two great forms, the Talmud of Babylon, and that of Jerusalem. The former is the more important, and is more learned and mystical.

Among the tracts referred to, are: *Pirke Aboth*, PRQI ABUT, Sayings of the Fathers; *Baba Kama*, BBA QMA, The first Gate; *Baba Bathra*, BBA BTRA, The Latter Gate; *Baba Metsia*, BBA MTzIOA, The Middle Gate. The work *Schaare Orah* mentioned by Rosenroth is the Hebrew ShOR AURH or Gate of Light written by Rabbi Joseph Gikatilla ben Abraham. The *Liber Pardes* of Rosenroth is the book *Sepher Pardesh Rimmonim*, or Garden of Pomegranates, its author was Rabbi Moses Cordovero, or Remak, who flourished about 1550. The value of this treatise is so largely dependent upon the Literal Kabalah and the method of Gematria, or the mutual conversion between letters and numbers that it is wise to introduce here a table of the English letters attributed to the Hebrew Letters and Numbers.

The system followed is that conventional one laid down in Wynn Westcott on "Numbers", which has also been adopted in each of the previous volumes of the series of *Collectanea Hermetica*. The system is only an approximation to the true rendering of Hebrew into English; as for example I is adopted for Yod, but some authors used I or Y orJ; and for Ayin, O is adoped which has sometimes the force of Ay and O, and at others of Gn, when used as a consonant.

Aleph A 1 Vau V 6 Kaph K 20 Ayin O 70 Shin Sh 300

Beth B 2 Zain Z 7 Lamed L 30 Peh P 80 Tau T 400

Gimel G 3 Cheth Ch 8 Mem M 40 Tzaddi Tz 90

Daleth D 4 Teth Th 9 Nun N 50 Qoph Q 100

Heh H 5 Yod I 10 Samech S 60 Resh R 200

The special final Letters are not used as numerals in the *Aesh Metzareph*. The *Aesh Metzareph* is almost entirely Alchymical in its teachings, and is suggestive rather than explanatory in its words. The allegorical method of teaching runs through it, and the similes have to be kept carefully in mind, otherwise confusion will result. Several Alchymic processes are set out, but not in such a way that they could be carried out by a neophyte; any attempt to do so would discover that something vital was missing at one stage or other. But although the *Aesh Metzareph* is not a manual of practical Alchymy, yet an attentive study of its statements considered with accurate relation to the numerical allusions, may give some true conclusions as to the materia and agents to be employed in the several forms of Transmutation. The nominal Christian of narrow views will see in this tract a confirmation of his opinion, that Alchymy is an unholy art and prompted by the Evil One; and there is perhaps no book which contains more Scripture verses referred to as illustrating the means and aims of Alchymy; so that perhaps such a one may point to this work as the brightest example of the assertion that "the Devil can quote even Holy Scripture to his purpose."

APPENDIX SEVEN

(original spelling has been kept throughout)

CHAPTER ONE: AESCH MEZAREPH, PURIFYING FIRE.

A CHYMICO-KABALISTIC TREATISE, COLLECTED FROM THE KABALA DENUDATA OF KNORR VON ROSENROTH. *Translated by a Lover of Philalethes, 1714.*

Elisha was a most notable prophet, an example of natural wisdom, a despiser of riches, (as the history of the healing of Naaman showeth, 2 Kings, c.5, v.16) and therefore truly rich. According to what is said in Pirke Aboth, viz., Who is rich ? He that rejoiceth in his portion, cap. 4. For so the true physician of impure metals hath not an outward show of riches, but is rather like the Tohu of the first Nature, empty and void. Which word is of equal number with the word Elisha, viz., 411. For it is a very true saying in Baba Kama, fol. 71. col. 2. The thing which causeth riches, (such as natural wisdom) is supplied instead of riches.

Learn therefore to purify Naaman, coming from the north, out of Syria, and acknowledge the power of Jordan: Which is as it were Jar-din that is the River of Judgment flowing out of the north.

And remember that which is said in Baba Bathra, fol. 25, col. 2. He that will become wise, let him live in the South; and he that will grow rich, let him turn himself toward the north, etc. Although in the same place Rabbi Joshua Ben Levi says, let him live always in the south, for whilst be becomes wise, at the same time he becomes rich. "Length of Days is in her right hand, and in her left, Riches and Honour." Prov., c.3, v.16. So thou wilt not desire other riches.

But know, that the mysteries of this wisdom, differ not from the superior mysteries of the Kabalah. For such as is the consideration of the predicaments in holiness, the same is also in impurity; and the same Sephiroth which are in Atziluth, the same are in Assiah, yea, the same in that kingdom, which is commonly called the although their excellency is always greater upon the spiritual plane. Therefore the metallic root here possesseth the place of Kether, which hath an occult nature, involved in great obscurity, and from which all metals have their origin; even as the nature of Kether is hidden, and the other Sephiroth flow from thence.

Lead hath the place of Chokmah, because Chokmah immediately proceeds from Kether, as it immediately comes from the metallic root, and in enigmatic similes, it is called the "father" of the following natures.

Tin possesseth the place of Binah, shewing age, by its greyness, and shadowing forth severity and judicial rigour, by its crackling.

Silver is placed under the Classis of Chesed, by all the masters of the Kabalah, chiefly for its colour and use.

Thus far the white natures. Now follow the red.

Gold is placed under Geburah, according to the most common opinion of the Kabalists; Job in c.37, v.22, also tells us that gold cometh from the north, not only for its colour, but for the sake of its heat and sulphur.

Iron is referred to Tiphereth, for he is like a man of war, according to Exod., c.15, v.2, and hath the name of "Seir Anpin", from his swift anger, according to Psalm 2, v.ult., "kiss the son lest he be angry."

Netzach and Hod are the two median places of the body, and the seminal receptacles, and refer to the hermaphroditic brass. So also the two pillars of the Temple of Solomon (referring to these two Sephiroth) were made of brass, I Kings, c.7, v.15.

Jesod is argent vive. For to this, the name "living" is characteristically given; and this living water is in every case the foundation of all Nature and of the metallic art.

But the true medicine of metals is referred to Malkuth, for many reasons; because it represents the rest of the natures under the metamorphoses of Gold and Silver, right and left, judgment and mercy, concerning which we will speak more largely elsewhere.

Thus I have delivered to thee the key to unlock many secret gates, and have opened the door to the inmost adyta of Nature. But if anyone hath placed those things in another order, I shall not contend with him, inasmuch as all systems tend to the one truth.

For it may be said, the three supernals are the three fountains of metallic things. The thick water is Kether, salt is Chokmah, and sulphur is Binah; for known reasons. And so the seven inferior will represent the seven metals, viz., Gedulah and Geburah, Silver and Gold; Tiphereth, Iron; Netzach and Hod, Tin and Copper; Jesod, Lead; and Malkuth will be the metallic woman, and the Luna of the wise men; and the field into which the seeds of secret minerals ought to be cast, that is the water of Gold, as this name (Mezahab) occurs, Genesis, c.36, v.39.

But know, my Son, that such mysteries are hid in these things as no tongue may be permitted to utter. But I will not offend any more with my tongue, but will keep my mouth with a bridle, Psalm 39, v.2.

Gehazi the Servant of Elisha, is the type of the vulgar students of Nature, who contemplate the valley and depths of Nature, but do not penetrate into her secrets.

Hence they labour in vain, and remain servants forever. They give counsel about procuring the son of the wise men whose generation exceeds the power of Nature, but they can add nothing to assist in his generation, 2 Kings, c.4, v.14 (for which purpose a man like Elisha is required). For Nature doth not open her secrets to them, v.26, but contemns them, v.30, and the raising of the dead is impossible to them, v.31. They are covetous, cap. 5, v.20; liars, v.22; deceivers, v.25; prattlers of other men's deeds, 2 Kings, c.8, v.4-5, and instead of riches, contract a leprosy themselves, that is disease, contempt and poverty, v.27. For the word Gehazi, and the word Chol, profane or common, have both the same number.

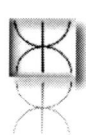

ILLUSTRATIONS

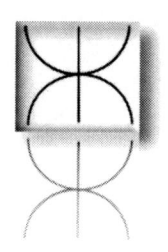

Figure One: The Tree of Life

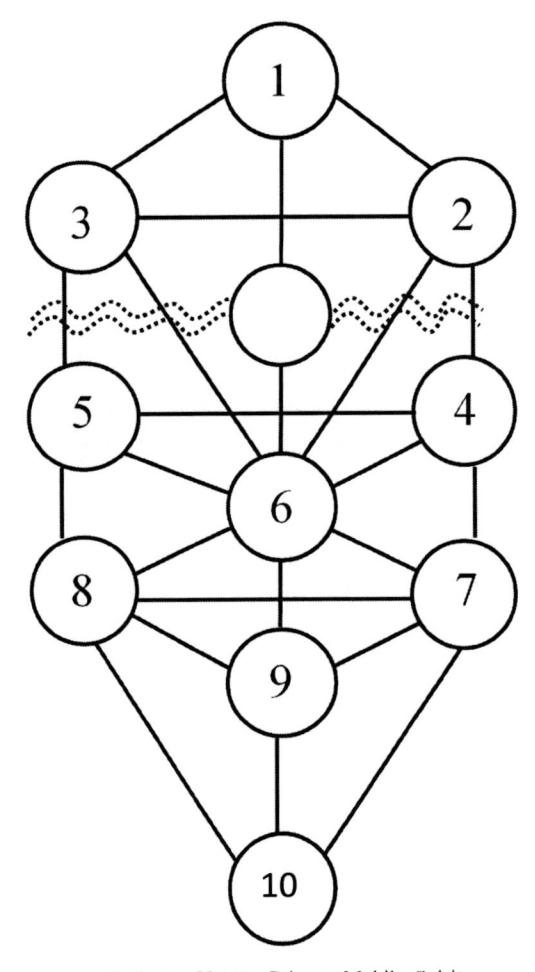

1: Crown, Uranus, Primum Mobile, Spirit
2: Wisdom, Neptune, Zodiac or Star Father
3: Understanding, Saturn, Great Mother
4: Mercy, Jupiter, Expansion, Giving and Creating
5: Severity, Mars, Reduction, Taking and Destroying
6: Beauty or Harmony, Sun, Balance
7: Victory, Venus, Feelings, Exaltation.
8: Glory, Mercury, Thought, Scintillation, Brilliance
9: Foundation, Moon and sub-lunar realm
10: Kingdom, Manifest Earth within sub-lunar realm.

Figure Two: The Three Worlds of Mon, Sun, Stars

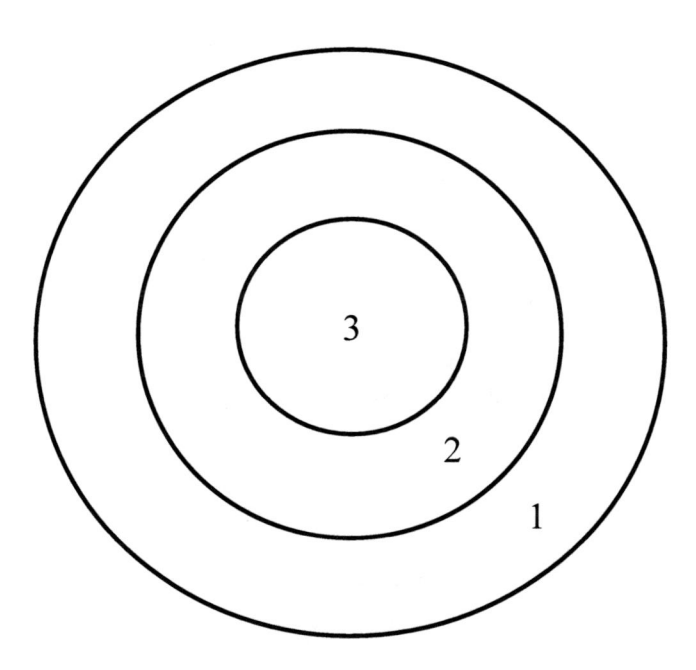

Key to Figure Two: envision as spheres.

1: Stellar Universe Enfolds Solar System

2: Solar System Enfolds Moon and Earth

3: Moon and Earth and all Earthly Nature

Figure Three: Seven Planetary Spheres Enfolding

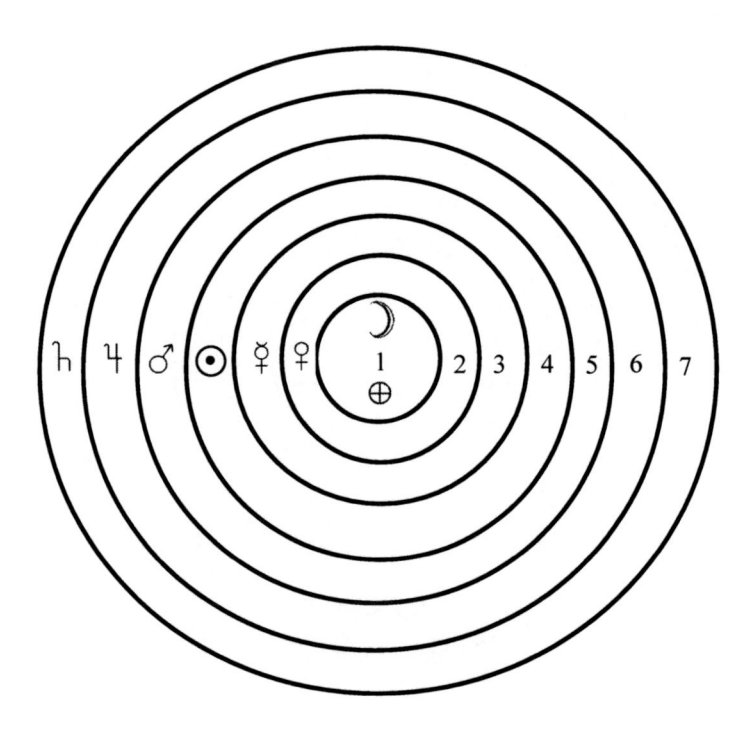

Key to Figure Three: envision as spheres

1: Earth/Moon
2: Venus
3: Mercury
5: Mars
6: Jupiter
7: Saturn

Figure Four: The Sevenfold Directions

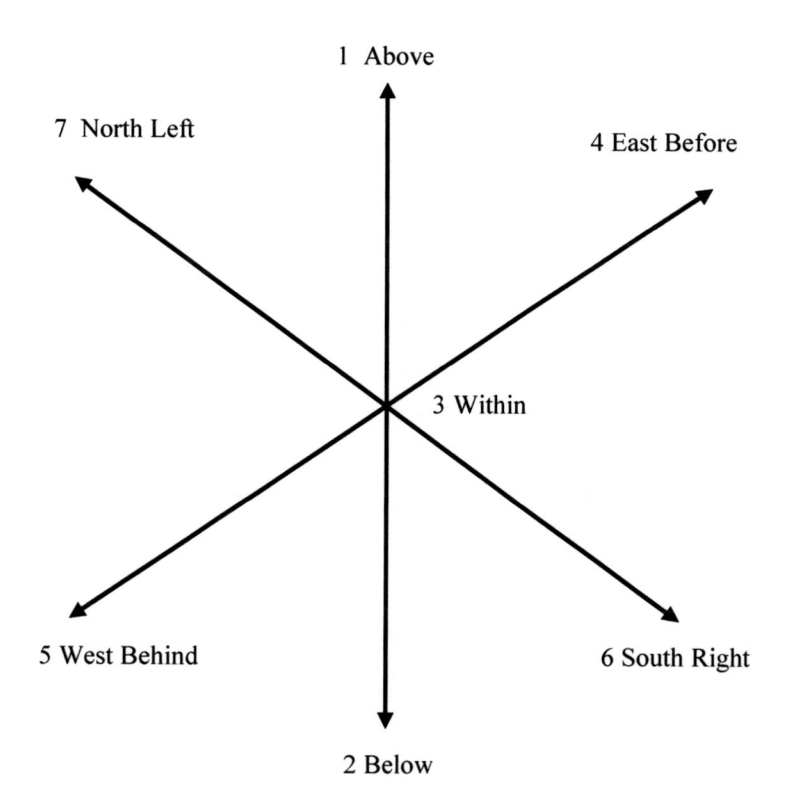

```
              1 Above
                ↑
7 North Left         4 East Before
   ↖                    ↗
         3 Within
   ↙                    ↘
5 West Behind        6 South Right
                ↓
              2 Below
```

The Seven Directions

Human: 1 Above/2 Below/3 Within/4 Before/5 Behind/6 Right/7 Left.

Environmental: 1 Stars (above)/2 Underworld (below)/3 Land (surface)/4 East/5 West/6 South/7 North

Figure Five: The Interaction Point

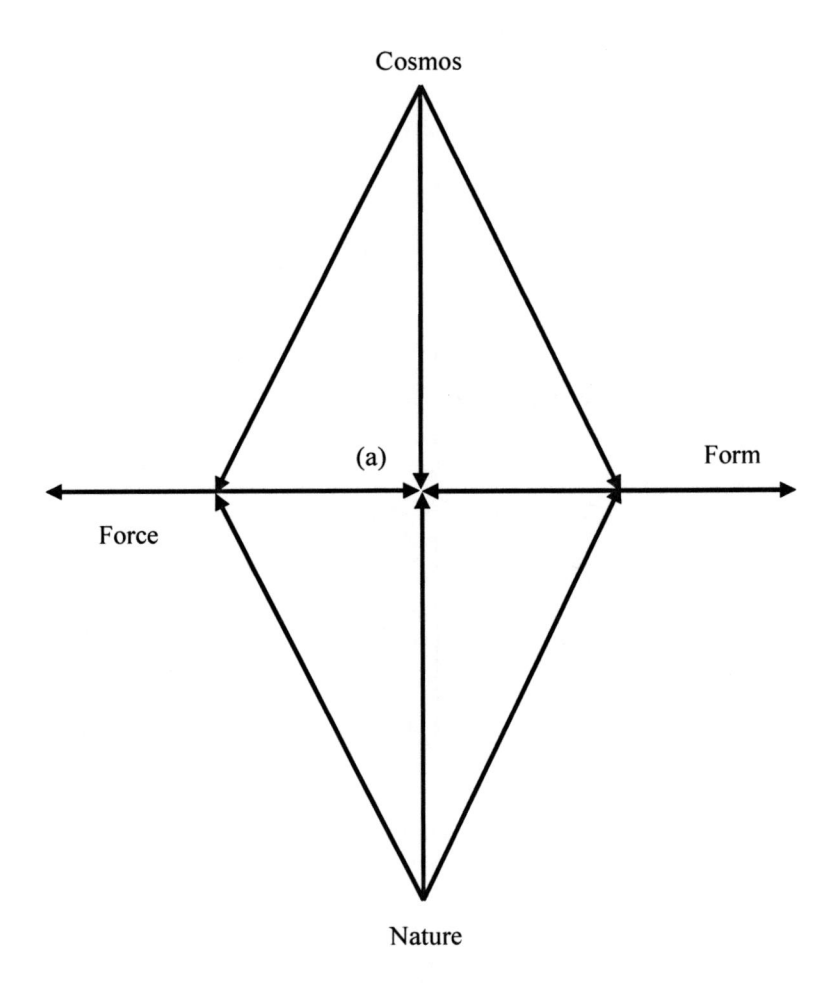

Cosmos

(a)

Force

Form

Nature

Figure Six: The Rising Earth Light becomes the Red and White Dragons

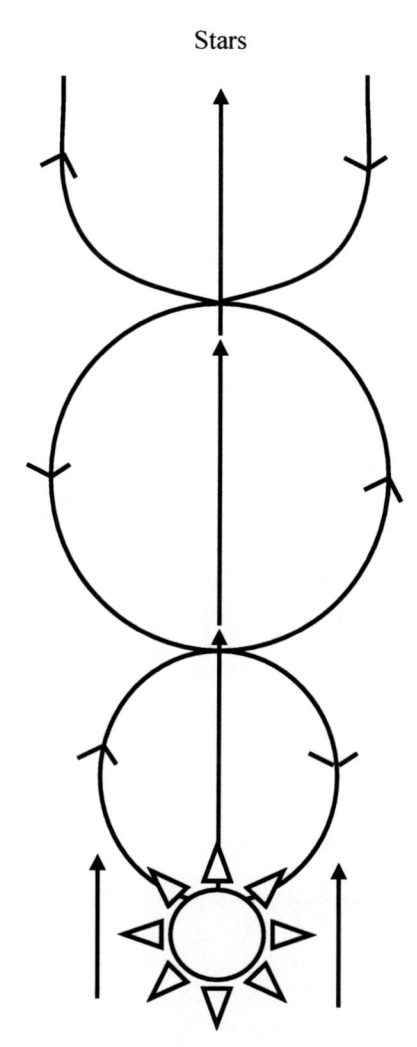

Stars

Rising Earth Light

Figure Seven: Four Archangels Upon the Tree of Life

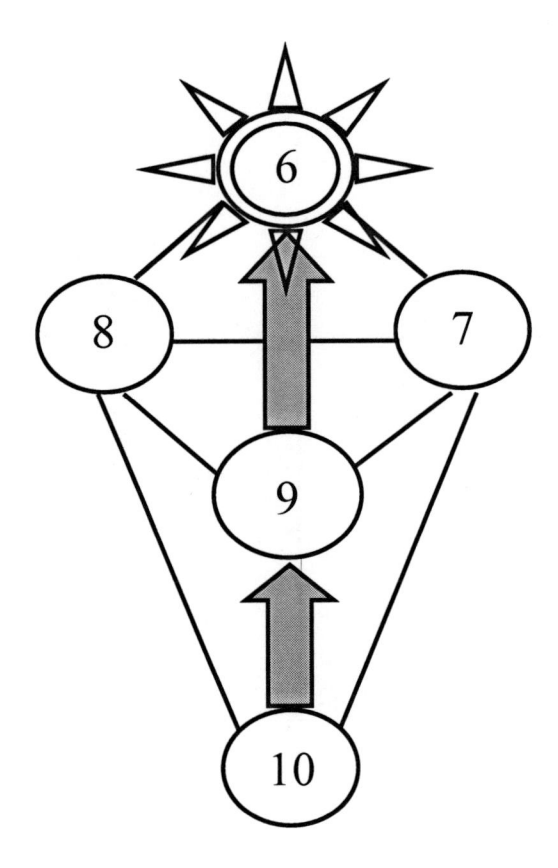

Key to Figure Seven

6: Michael / Sun
7: Auriel / Venus
8: Raphael / Mercury
9: Gabriel / Moon
10: Manifest World / Earth

Figure Eight: The Three Wheels

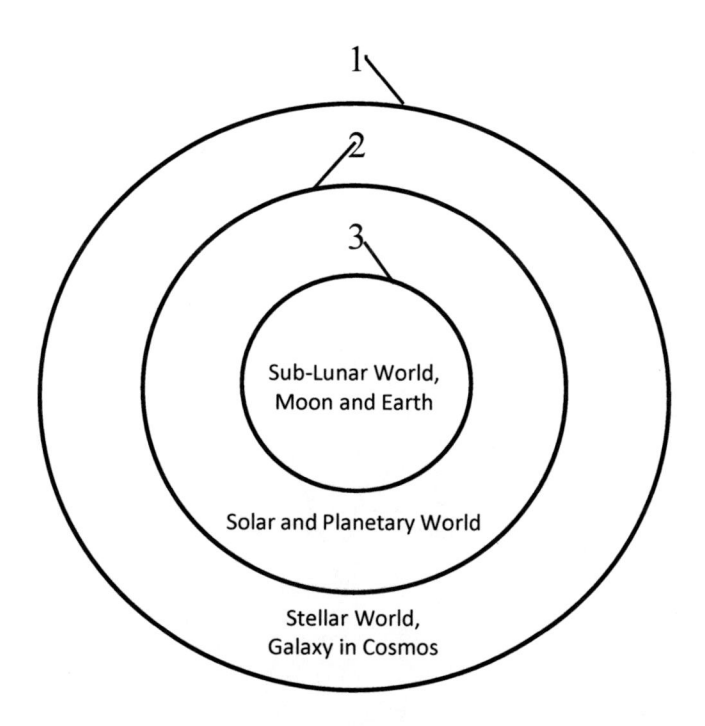

1
2
3

Sub-Lunar World,
Moon and Earth

Solar and Planetary World

Stellar World,
Galaxy in Cosmos

Key to Figure Eight

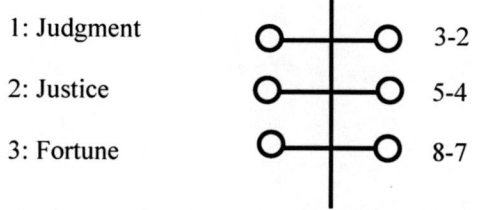

1: Judgment   O——O   3-2

2: Justice   O——O   5-4

3: Fortune   O——O   8-7

The Wheels of *Judgment, Justice* and *Fortune* are three nested spheres. The horizontal Paths on the Tree of Life are indicators or guide-lines for each enfoldment or sphere.

Figure Nine: The Three Vessels

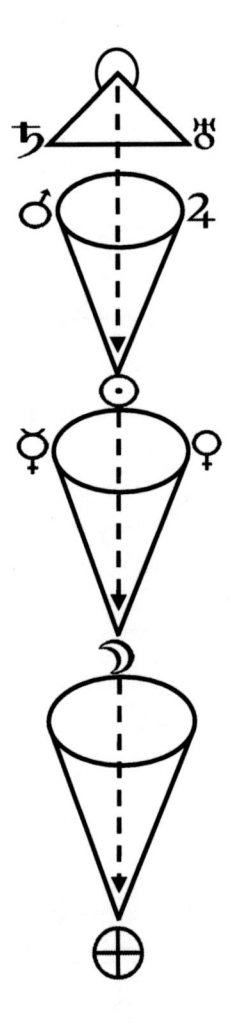

Figure Ten: The Triplicities

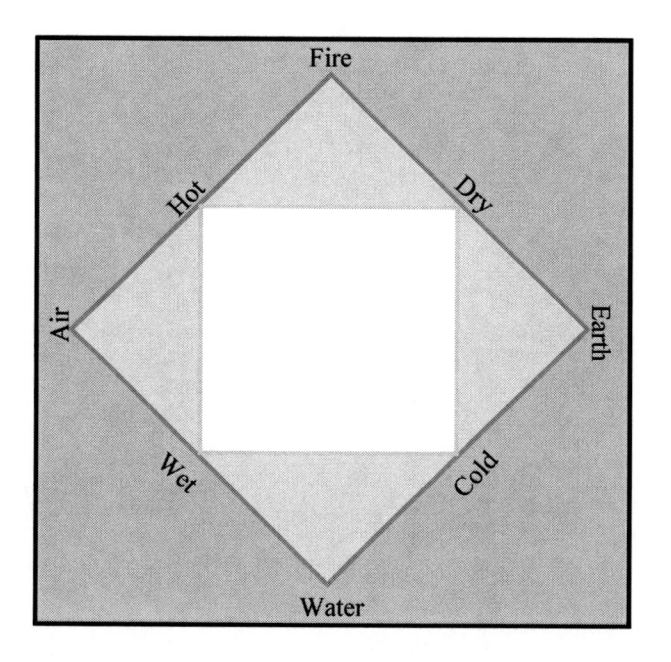

Figure Eleven: The Wheel of Life

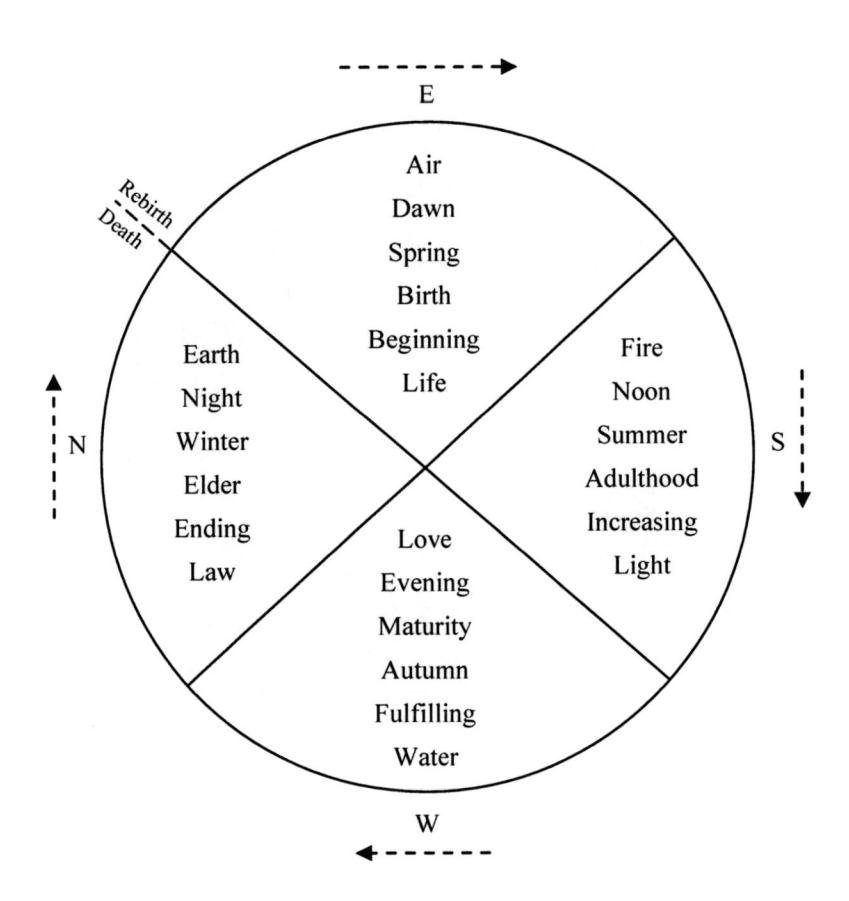

```
                    E →

                   Air
                   Dawn
                   Spring
                   Birth
         Earth    Beginning    Fire
         Night      Life       Noon
   N ↑   Winter                Summer   ↓ S
         Elder                 Adulthood
         Ending                Increasing
         Law       Love        Light
                   Evening
                   Maturity
                   Autumn
                   Fulfilling
                   Water

                    W ←
```

Rebirth / Death (NW)

Figure Twelve: The Pattern of the Vials

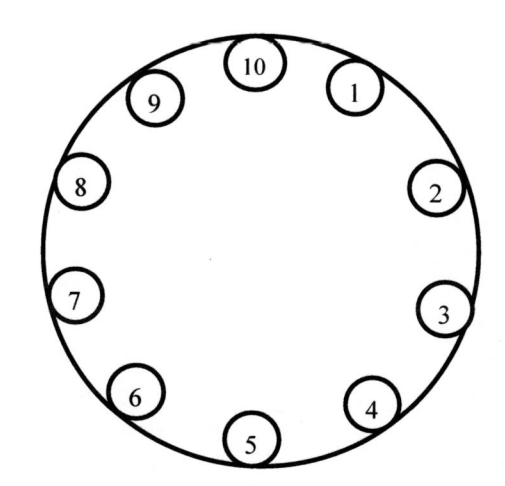

12.1

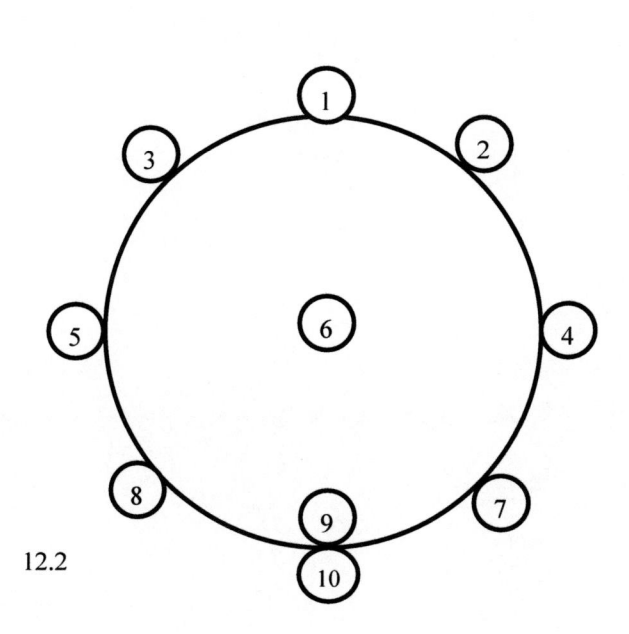

12.2

Figure Thirteen: Cord/Body

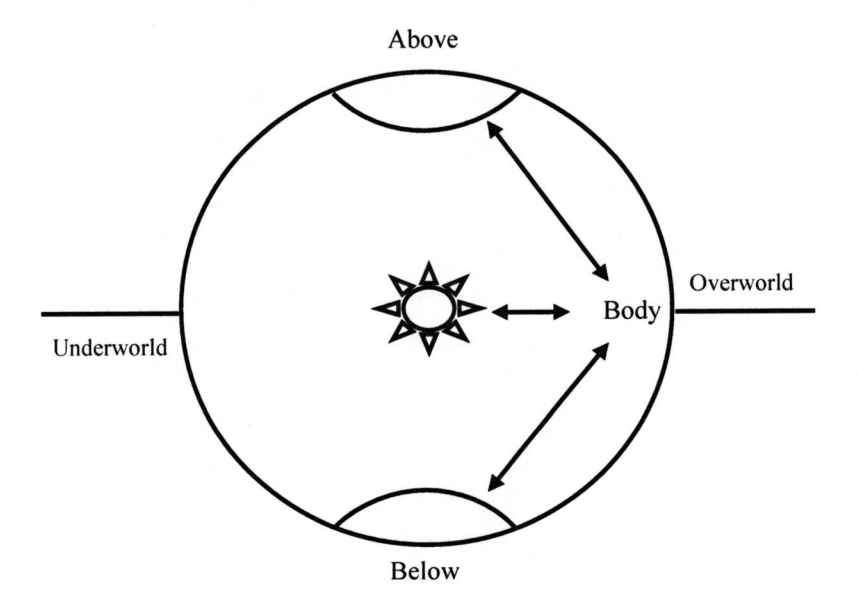

Figure Fourteen: The Four Holy Fires

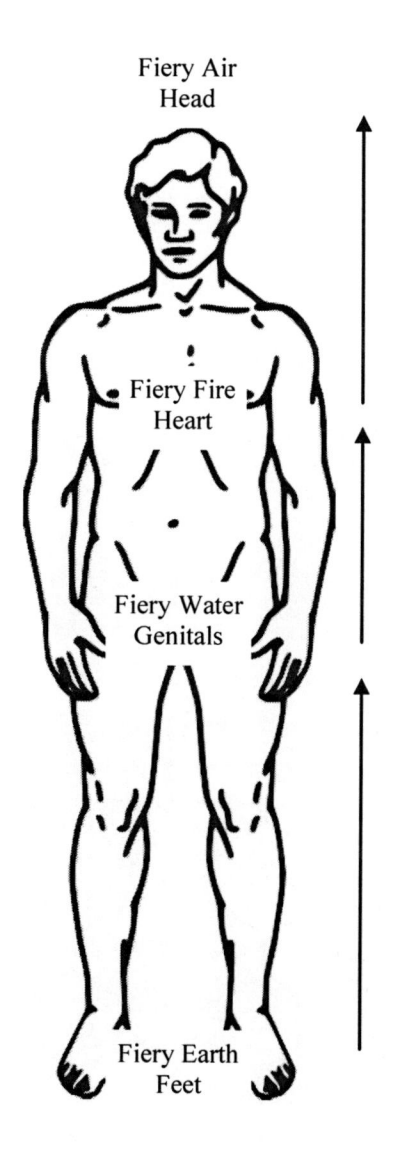

Fiery Air
Head

Fiery Fire
Heart

Fiery Water
Genitals

Fiery Earth
Feet

Figure Fifteen: Overworld and Underworld Tree

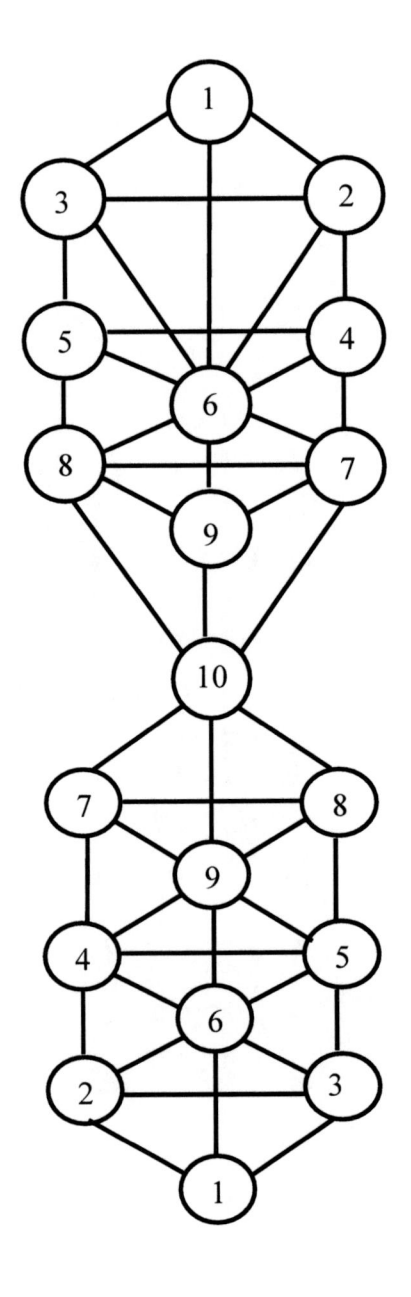

Figure Sixteen: Chaos and Eros

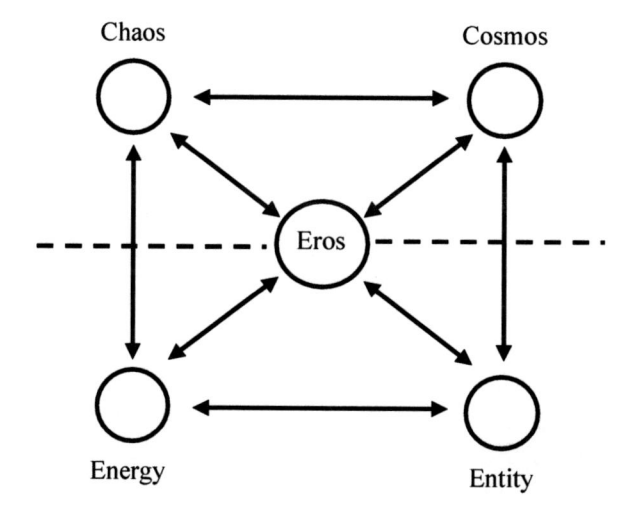

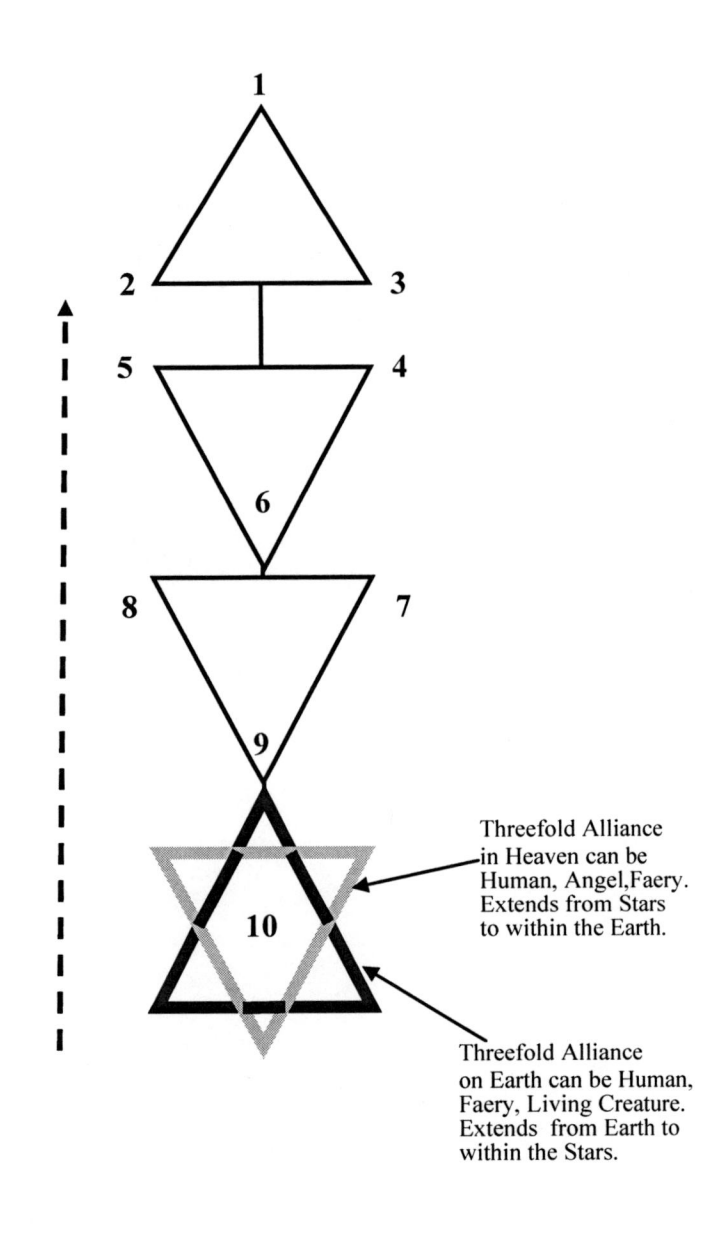

Figure Seventeen: Triads on the Tree of Life -
The Threefold Alliances

Threefold Alliance in Heaven can be Human, Angel, Faery. Extends from Stars to within the Earth.

Threefold Alliance on Earth can be Human, Faery, Living Creature. Extends from Earth to within the Stars.

Figure Eighteen: Long Triads on the Tree

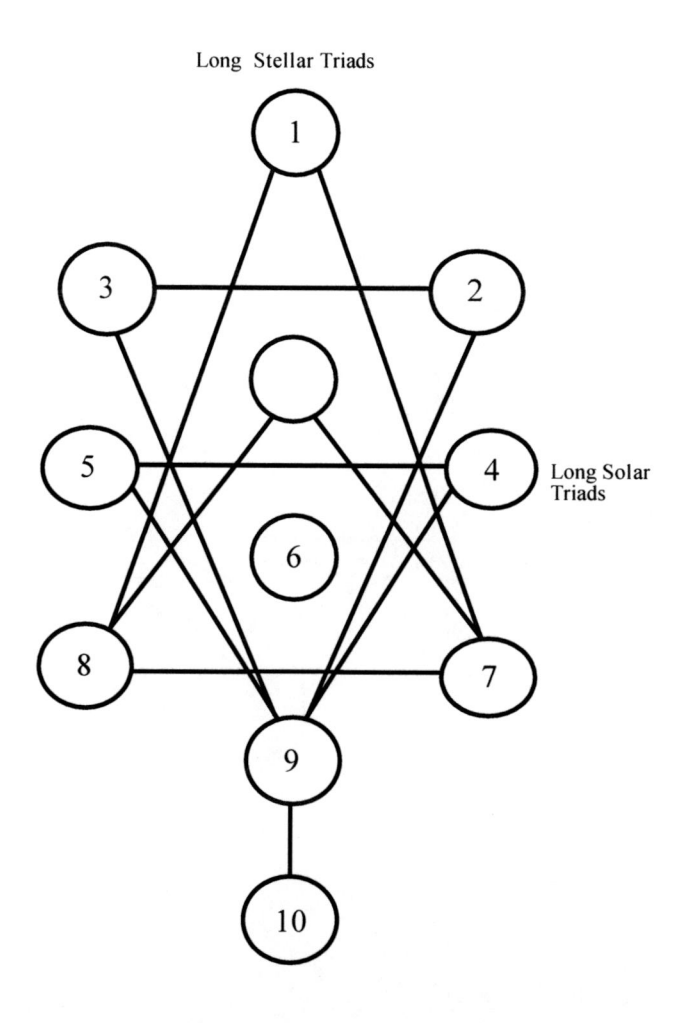

Long Stellar Triads

Long Solar Triads

1-7-8: Spirit, Feeling, Thought. [Uranus, Venus, Mercury] Sulphur, Copper, Quicksilver. Crown, Victory, Glory. *"Spirit Victorious and Radiant"*
2-3-9: Wisdom, Understanding, Foundation. [Neptune, Saturn, Moon] Salt, Lead, Silver. *"The Firmly Founded Vessel of Wisdom"*
4-5-9: Mercy, Severity, Foundation. [Jupiter, Mars, Moon]Tin, Iron, Silver. *"The Firmly Founded Vessel of Balance "*.
(0)-7-8: Knowledge, Feeling, Thought. [Pluto, Venus, Mercury] Fusion,Copper, Quicksilver. *"Knowledge, Victorious, and Radiant"* .

Figure Nineteen: Solar Emanations

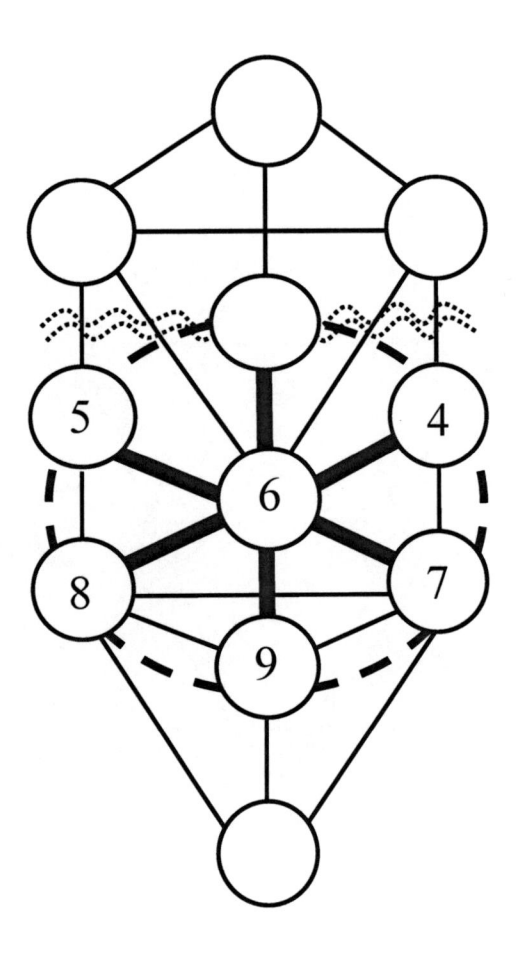

Figure Twenty: Nested Spheres

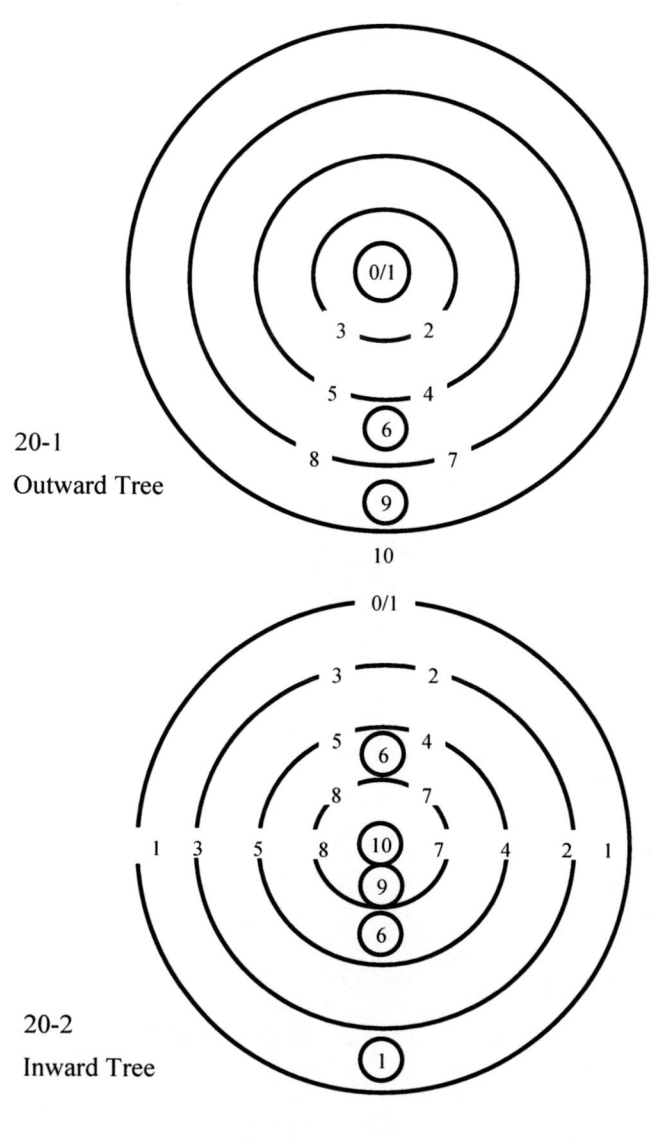

20-1
Outward Tree

20-2
Inward Tree

On Both Trees:
3-2 = 8-7
0-1 = 1-0
5-4 = 5-4

8+7 = 15 / 3+2 = 15

Figure Twenty-One: Progression of Angels

Fourfold — Holy Creatures

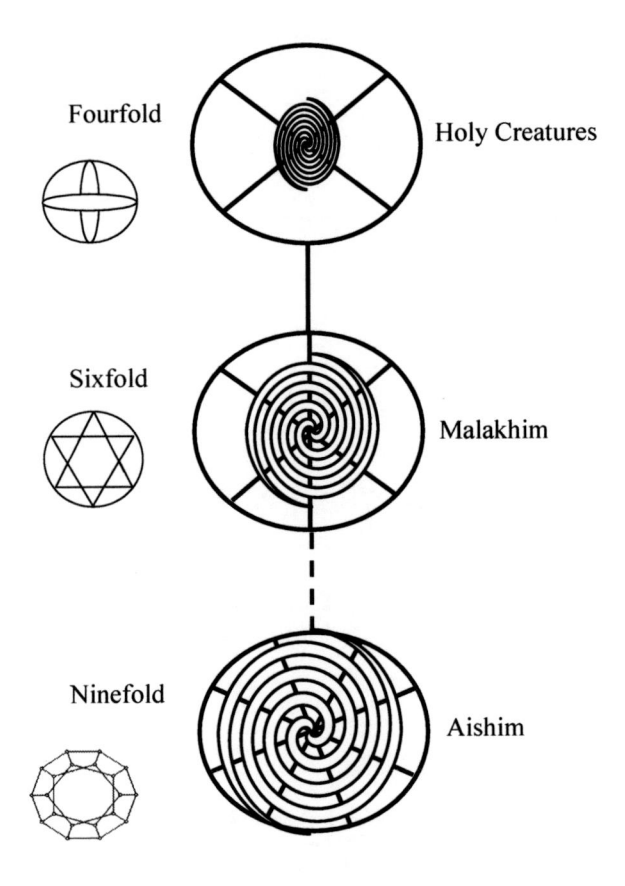

Sixfold — Malakhim

Ninefold — Aishim

The Manifesting Nature of the Four Elements or Roots of Creation. The *Holy Creatures* create the Sixfold Nature of the Sun and the *Malakhim*, that generate the Ninefold Nature of the Moon, the *Aishim*, that manifest the world of Nature. Our planet Earth is also Fourfold, through the Four *Kerubim* that embody Elemental power in Nature.

Figure Twenty-Two: Eight Sigils

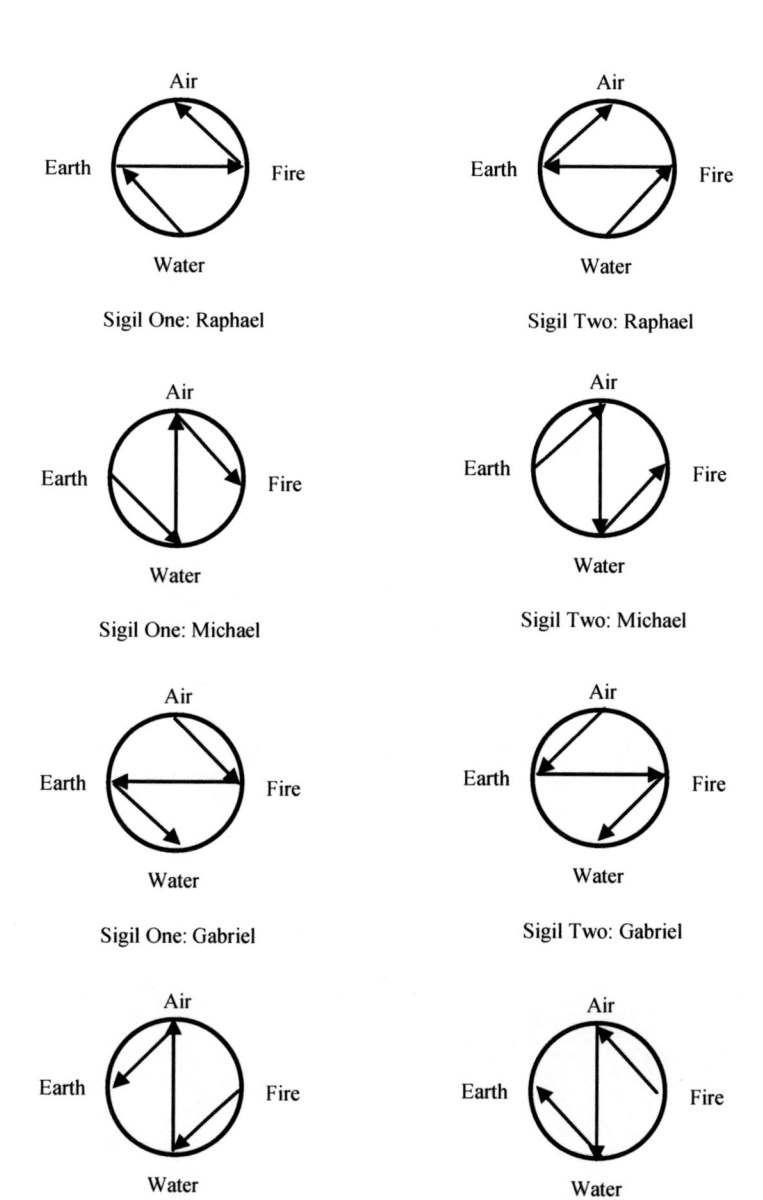

Sigil One: Raphael

Sigil Two: Raphael

Sigil One: Michael

Sigil Two: Michael

Sigil One: Gabriel

Sigil Two: Gabriel

Sigil One: Auriel

Sigil Two: Auriel

Figure Twenty-Three: Archangels and Angels upon the Tree of Life

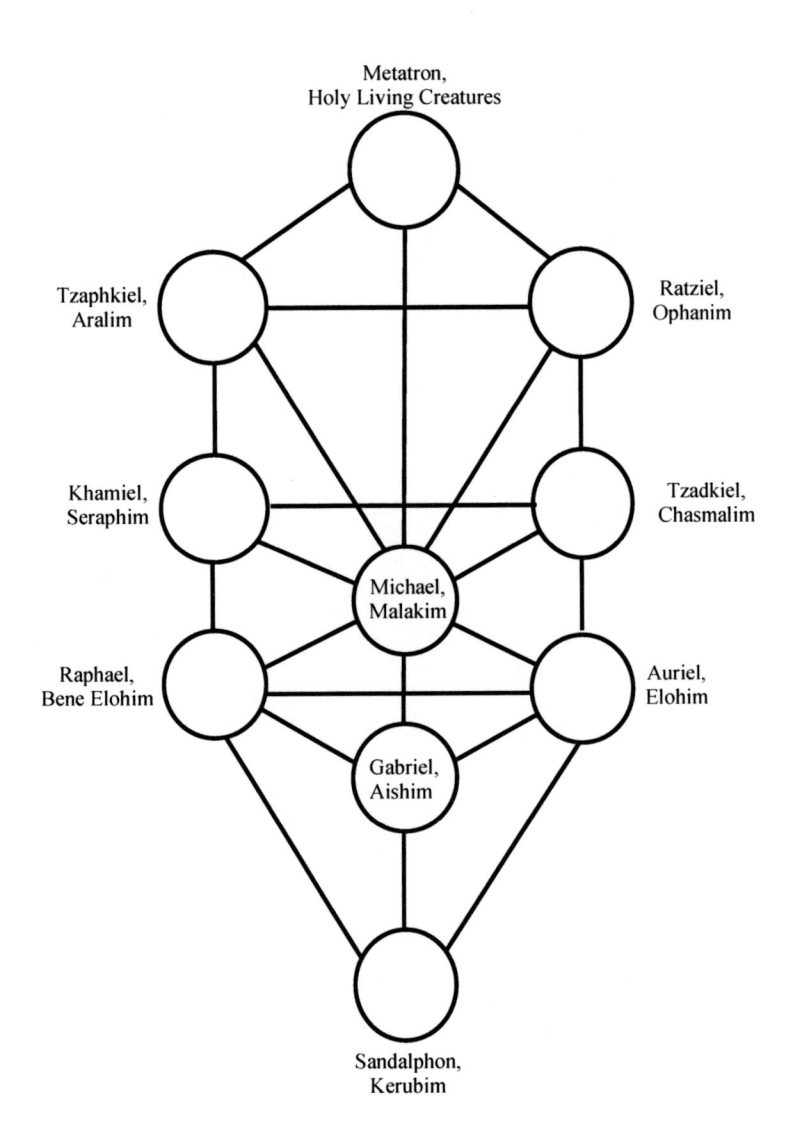

- Metatron, Holy Living Creatures
- Tzaphkiel, Aralim
- Ratziel, Ophanim
- Khamiel, Seraphim
- Tzadkiel, Chasmalim
- Michael, Malakim
- Raphael, Bene Elohim
- Auriel, Elohim
- Gabriel, Aishim
- Sandalphon, Kerubim

Figure Twenty-Four: Turning About the Wheel

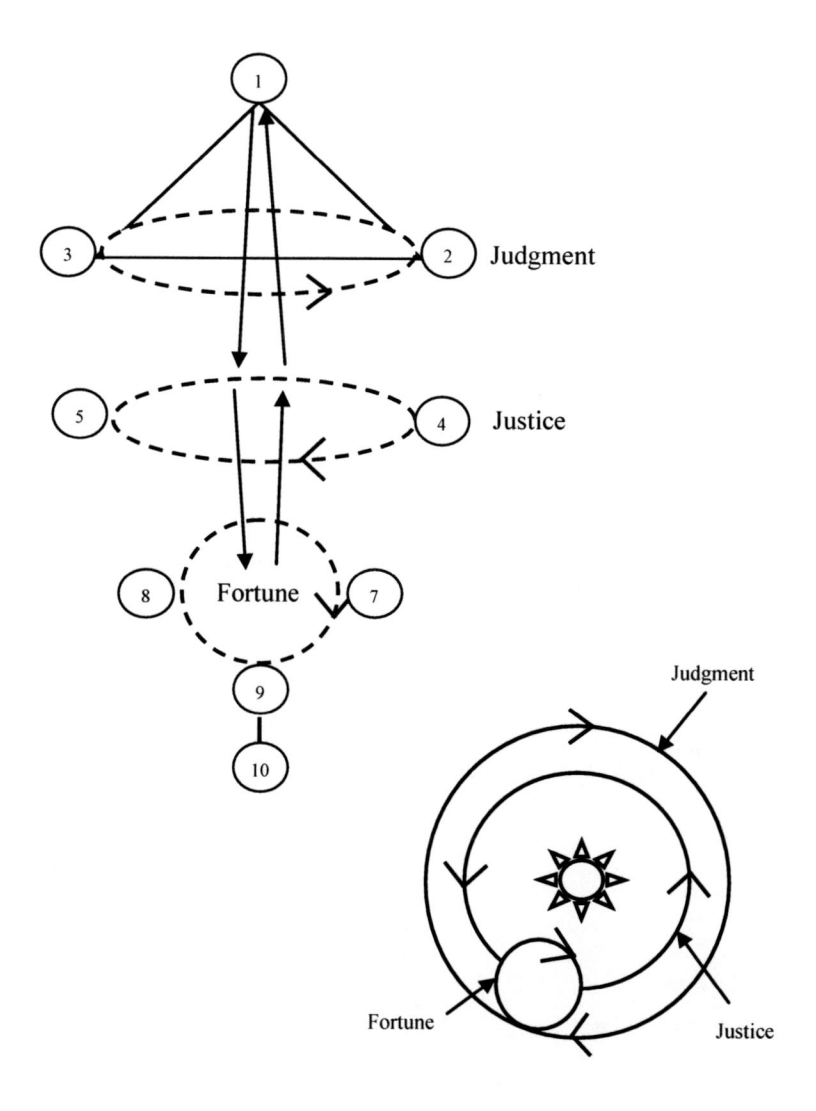

Figure Twenty Five: OverWorld - UnderWorld

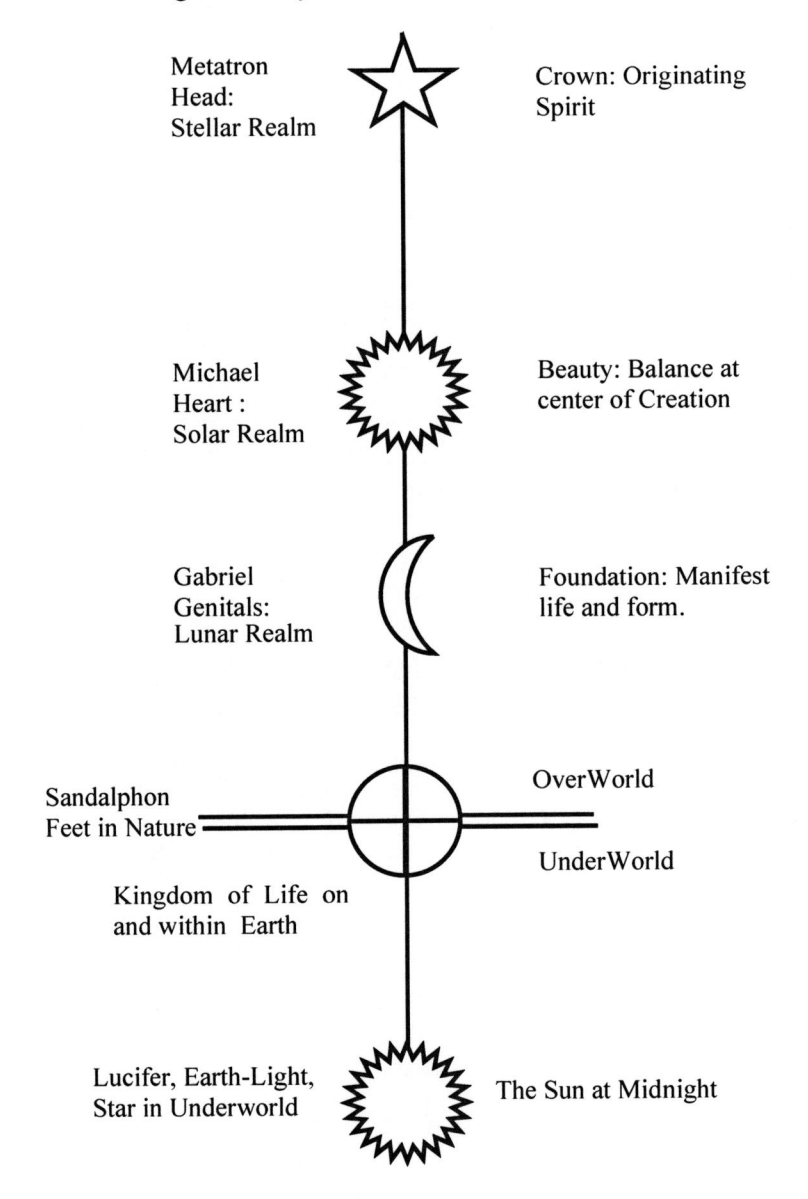

Metatron
Head:
Stellar Realm

Crown: Originating Spirit

Michael
Heart:
Solar Realm

Beauty: Balance at center of Creation

Gabriel
Genitals:
Lunar Realm

Foundation: Manifest life and form.

Sandalphon
Feet in Nature

OverWorld

UnderWorld

Kingdom of Life on and within Earth

Lucifer, Earth-Light,
Star in Underworld

The Sun at Midnight

The telluric fire of the planet is also stellar fire. The nearest Star is beneath our Feet. The Crown is in the Kingdom, in a different manner. Elevating the Metals reveals the Crown hidden within the Kingdom.

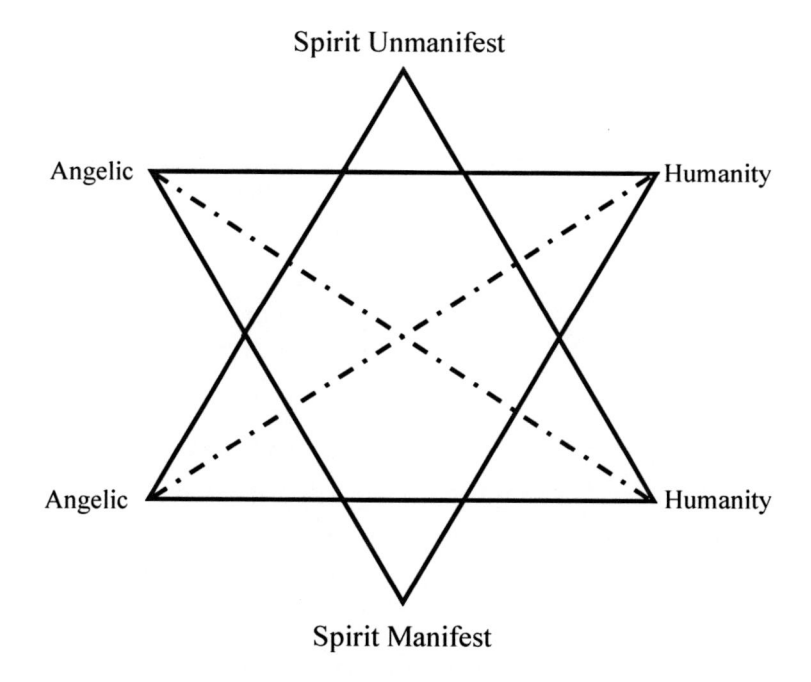

Figure Twenty Six: Hexagram and Pentagram

Figure Twenty Seven: Supernal Triad

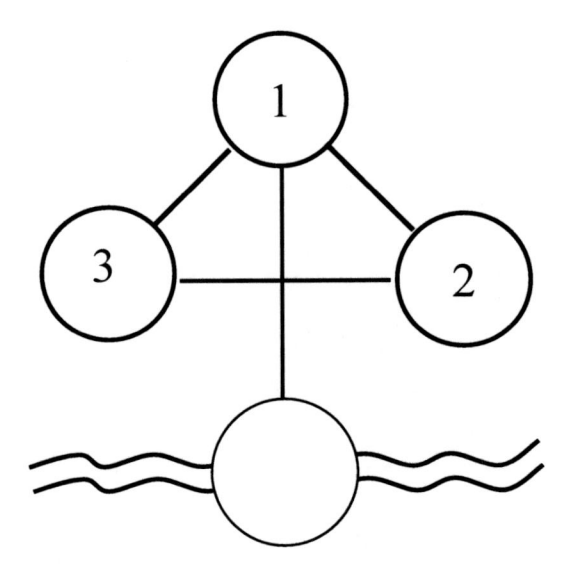

The Supernal Triad of Emanations: The spiritual powers of consciousness are Being, Wisdom, and Understanding. In mythic terms these are the mysterious divine source of Being, the Star Father, and the Great Mother. Further manifestations of the Tree of Life are reflections of this Triad.

Figure Twenty-Eight: Tree as Nested Spheres

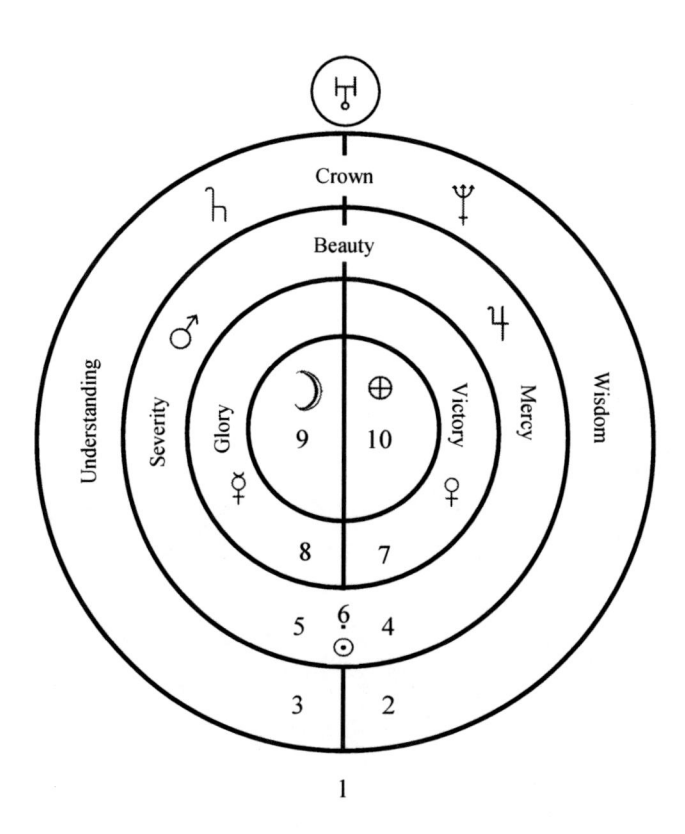

The Tree of Life is a Sphere, with many nested layers within it. The five nested spheres are the boundaries of the Four Spiritual Worlds of Origination, Creation, Formation, and Expression. They also contain the Three Manifest Worlds, of Stars, Sun and Planets, Moon and Earth.

Figure Twenty Nine: Elemental Tree of Life

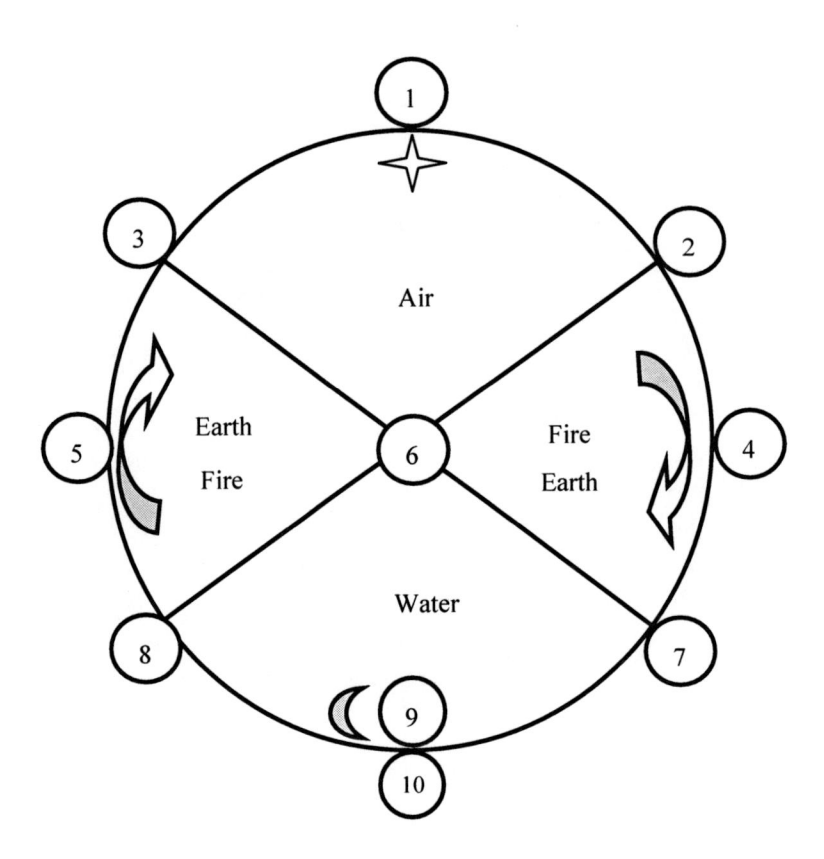

Figure Thirty: Reconciling the Worlds

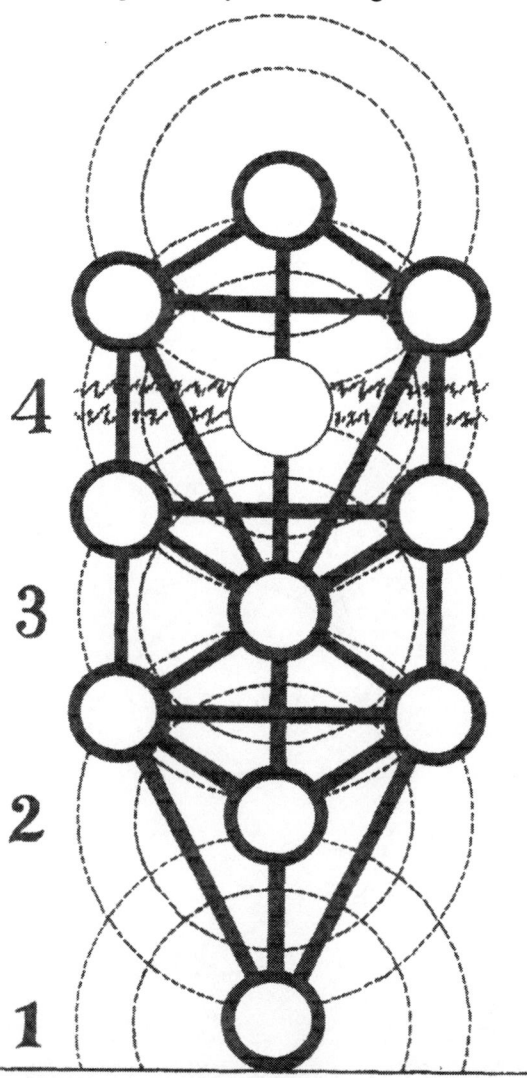

The four phases of Origination, Creation, Formation, and Expression, are often called the Four Worlds. This fourfold concept can be integrated with the Three Worlds of the physical and metaphysical cosmos, which are the Stellar, Solar, and Lunar Worlds, embracing the Ten Emanations. The Stellar World links the fields of Origination and Creation, the Solar World (our Solar System) links the fields of Creation and Formation (for us), and the Lunar World (our Earth-Moon interaction) links the fields of Formation and Expression (here on Earth).

Figure Thirty One The Multifold Tree of Life

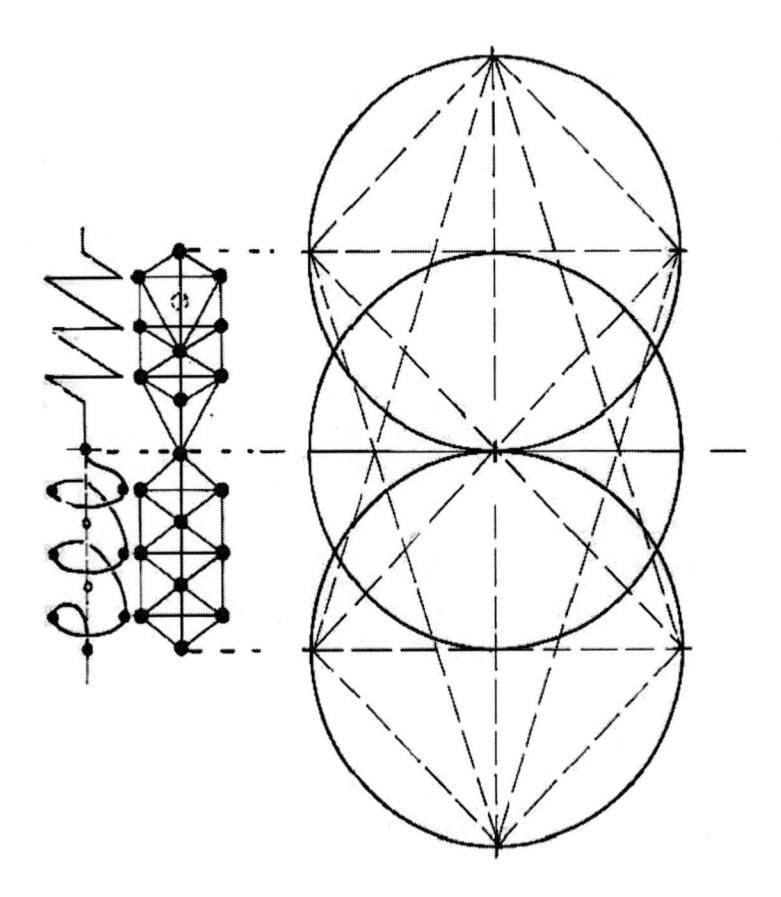

The Multifold Tree of Life as drawn by the Author in communion with Inner Contacts in 1973. This conceptual model led to insights and three-fold illustrations found in later books, including The UnderWorld Initiation, The Complete Merlin Tarot., and the Dreampower Tarot.

The Sphere of Art practice brings the upper and lower sphere together merging as one within the central sphere.

Figure Thirty Two: Threefold Tree of Life

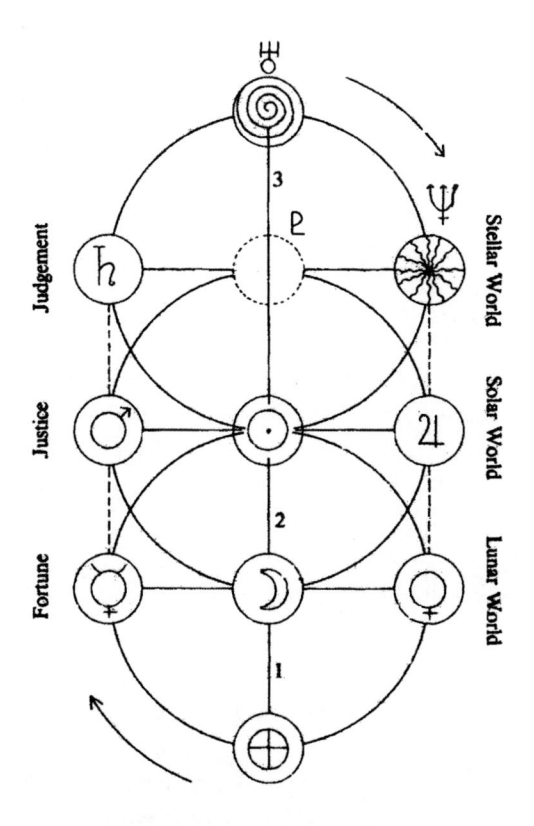

The Three Worlds and Three Wheels of the Tree of Life. Original drawing by the Author, 1978. Later incorporated into The Merlin Tarot.

AFTERWORD

This book has a numerical Qabalistic structure, in the number of pages, chapters, appendices, and illustrations. The illustrations may be used as a meditational or contemplative visionary sequence, in either direction, from 1-33, or from 33-1. This sequence may be undertaken at any time, either during the cycle of Elevation of the Materials, or in its own right. Eventually you will find that you have memorized the Illustrations, and that you can build them in your inner vision, without referring to a page. Most important of all, you will be able work *within* them as three-dimensional figures, gradually leading to other dimensions of awareness. At this stage, you will be able to work with the images within the Sphere of Art entirely from memory.

With the anonymous author of *Aesch Mezareph*, I can say: *Thus I have delivered to thee the key to unlock many secret gates, and have opened the door to the inmost adyta of Nature. But if anyone hath placed those things in another order, I shall not contend with him, inasmuch as all systems tend to the one truth.*

R J Stewart, Illinois, Imbolc, 2012

The Night is Dark,
The Way is Lost,
Not yet Forgotten,
Discover Light within Yourself,
Thus to Become a Lamp For Others.

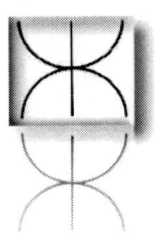

NOTES and REFERENCE SOURCES

To save space, some notes contain links to reference sources online. Such sources are sometimes ephemeral, but I have tried to select those that are substantial, have endurance, and that offer, in themselves, well researched references or complete texts.

1: Kaplan, Aryeh, *Sefer Yetzirah*, Weiser 1997

2: Stewart, R.J, *The Sphere of Art (Vol 1)*, R J Stewart Books 2008

3: Stewart, R.J. *Merlin, The Prophetic Vision and Mystic Life*, R. J. Stewart Books, 2009. (First published Penguin Arkana 1986 as two separate volumes). Also: Stewart R.J. *The Well of Light, from Faery Healing to Earth Healing, the Mystery of the Double Rose*. R J Stewart Books, 2007, and sections on the Evolutionary and Involutionary Streams and Dragons in (2).

4: Stewart, R.J. *Earth Light* and *Power Within the Land*, Mercury Publishing, 2002. First published Element Books, 1988. Also, *The Well of Light*, ibid.

5: Stewart, R.J. *The Merlin Tarot*, deck of images and book. Aquarian Press, 1988. Also The *Complete Merlin Tarot* Harper Collins 1992. Developed from proto-tarot images in the 12th century Merlin texts, by Geoffrey of Monmouth, deriving from Welsh bardic tradition. See also (3), *Merlin, The Prophetic Vision and Mystic Life*.

6: www.innerconvocation.com . Also: Stewart R.J. *The Inner Temples*, audio CD with original music, R J Stewart Books. www.rjstewart.net The original Inner Temples meditations can be found in (2) above.

7: *The Sanctuary of Avalon* is a small sanctuary of silence hidden among the trees on the slopes of Glastonbury Tor in Britain. A further sanctuary is located in the USA. Both sanctuaries and related activities such as training and community work in spiritual education are supported by tax-deductible charitable donations. For more information go to www.innerconvocation.com or contact rjspeak@earthlink.net, with "Sanctuary of Avalon" in the subject line.

8: Stewart, R.J., *Living Magical Arts* and *Advanced Magical Arts*, R J Stewart Books. LMA first published by Blandford Press, 1986. AMA first published by Element Books, 1989. Note: *any editions other than those of Element or R J Stewart Books are pirated* and contain many inaccuracies. Meditations, Ceremonies, and Visionary Workings from *Advanced Magical Arts*, with original music, are available as a 2 CD set from www.rjstewart.net

9 Kaplan, Aryeh, *Meditation and Kabbalah*, Weiser 1985.

10: Corbin, Henri, *Swedenborg and Esoteric Islam*. Swedenborg Foundation, 1995. Corbin once stated, of his early studies, "Platonism, expressed in terms of the Zoroastrian Angelogy of ancient Persia, illuminated the path that I was seeking."

11: Stewart, R. J. *The Miracle Tree, De-Mystifying the Qabalah*, New Page, 2002. The task for this book was set by W G Gray during the early 1970's when he advised that I would one day write a book that clarified Qabalistic methods into direct modern English. It took me almost thirty years before I felt ready to attempt the task, and the result was *The Miracle Tree*, with a companion CD of original Qabalistic meditations and music.

12: http://www.rexresearch.com/adept/aacont.htm is one of many comprehensive sources for alchemical texts currently available on the Internet. I do not necessarily support or endorse all of the opinions given on such sites, but respect the diligent work undertaken to freely provide alchemical historical reference material for all readers.

13: Stewart, R.J. *The Spirit Cord*, R J Stewart Books, 2007.

14: In his Introduction to (1) Aryeh Kaplan writes " The commentaries which treat *Sefer Yetzirah* as a theoretic text, read much of it in the third person: 'He combined', 'He formed,' and the like. According to this reading the text is referring to God's creation. In many cases, however, the grammatical form more closely resembles the imperative. The author is telling the reader to 'combine' and 'form' as if he was actually giving instructions. In many other cases the text is unambiguously instructive, as in such passages as, 'if your heart runs, return to the place,' and 'understand with wisdom, and be wise with understanding'." (Kaplan, Introduction, page x). This is a significant comment, and a powerful Qabalistic hint, regarding practice.

15: For a short article on the Platonic Solids, go to: http://en.wikipedia.org/wiki/Platonic_solid .
For many illustrations of Platonic Solids in various forms, go to http://www.google.com/search?q=Platonic+Solids .

16 For a clear brief article on remarkable geo-magnetic finds at Stanton Drew prehistoric alignments in Somerset, Britain, go to: http://www.ucl.ac.uk/prehistoric/past/past28.html#Stanton

17 Stewart, R.J. *Music and the Elemental Psyche* Aquarian Press, 1987 (also titled) *The Spiritual Dimensions of Music* Destiny books, 1990. An audio CD, *Calling in the Elements*, of Elemental Calls and Sound Shapes, plus a guided visualization, is available from www.rjstewart.net

18 Achad, Frater, (Charles Stanfield Jones) *The Anatomy of the Body of God* . A PDF edition of this out-of-copyright book can be found at http://hermetic.com/achad/pdf/anatomy.pdf . While I do not necessarily endorse or follow the beliefs and practices developed by Frater Achad, *The Anatomy of the Body of God* is a striking example of early 20th century original Qabalistic insight, written at a time when most books merely copied standard Tree of Life illustrations from the ground-breaking works of the great Victorian adepts.

19 http://en.wikipedia.org/wiki/Christian_Knorr_von_Rosenroth offers a short biography of the life and work of Knorr von Rosenroth, a 17th century European Hebraist and mystical scholar who translated a number of significant Kabbalistic works, including *Aesch Mezareph*. See also Addendum C, on the compendium of *Kabbalah Denudata* : http://www.digital-brilliance.com/kab/karr/ccineb.pdf . The main document of this PDF is a very comprehensive and well researched set of references, with some commentary, on sources and translations for Christian Qabalah, and therefore of a large number of historical Qabalistic/Kabbalistic sources.

20 http://aleph500.huji.ac.il/nnl/dig/books/bk001091404.html leads to a full digitized copy of *Kabbalah Denudata* photographed from an original edition, including the remarkable Kabbalistic illustrations.

21 Westcott, W. Wynn, *Aesch Mezareph*, page 57.

22 Westcott, A.M. Preface, page 6.

23 http://en.wikipedia.org/wiki/Obed-Edom gives the Biblical references without any critical analysis or interpretation.

24 Westcott, A.M. , note 19, page 47. He refers the note to Frater Q.S.N, i.e. himself, *Quod Scis Nescis* .

25 Westcott, A.M. note 31,page 50: *The Magic Square given is not the true Square of Sol. This word QMIO, commonly written Kamea, is a Mystical Square, sub-divided into lesser squares by perpendicular and horizontal lines; in each space is placed a number or equivalent letter or letters, so arranged as to give the same total by addition in each line, up and down, or across.* Westcott offers another square, which, he says, is the standard Kamea for Sol or Gold. A detailed article on the history and construction of Magic Squares from a mathematical perspective can be found at: http://en.wikipedia.org/wiki/Magic_square

26: For an annotated translation of *Baba Bathra* see : www.come-and hear.com/bababathra/bababathra_0.html#intro

27: This famous quote is seldom given in full. It comes from the Babylonian *Talmud*, tractate Shabbos 31a . "On another occasion it happened that a certain heathen came before Shammai and said to him, "Make me a proselyte, on the condition that you teach me the whole Torah while I stand on one foot." Thereupon he chased him away with the builder's cubit that was in his hand. When he came before Hillel, (and asked him to teach the entire Torah while standing on one foot) Hillel replied, "What is hateful to you, do not do to your neighbor: that is the whole Torah while the rest is commentary; go and learn it."

28: This process is described by Kaplan in his Introduction to *Sefer Yetzirah* (revised edition, Weiser, 1997) pp xvii-xviii.

29: http://www.sacred-texts.com/jud/t06/index.htm links to a translation of the Babylonian Talmud.

30: Another interpretation that is sometimes proposed, is based on *physical* Alchemy and mundane chemistry, which is that the "thick water" used for the fire over water demonstrations was *naphtha*. This is suggested in II Maccabees, Ch 1, v 19-22.

31: The full quote from Proverbs 3 is as follows: 13 Happy is the man that findeth wisdom, and the man that getteth understanding. 14 For the merchandise of it is better than the merchandise of silver, and the gain thereof than fine gold.15 She is more precious than rubies: and all the things thou canst desire are not to be compared unto her.16 Length of days is in her right hand; and in her left hand riches and honour.17 Her ways are ways of pleasantness, and all her paths are peace.18 She is a tree of life to them that lay hold upon her: and happy is every one that retaineth her.19 The Lord by wisdom hath founded the earth; by understanding hath he established the heavens.20 By his knowledge the depths are broken up, and the clouds drop down the dew.21 My son, let not them depart from thine eyes: keep sound wisdom and discretion:22 So shall they be life unto thy soul, and grace to thy neck.23 Then shalt thou walk in thy way safely, and thy foot shall not stumble.

32: Westcott, A.M. note 18, page 47.

33: See (3) above for the telluric energy experiments of Luis Rota and Karl Schappeller that were researched by A R Heaver in the 1930's

34: Gray, W.G. *Magical Ritual Methods*, Helios , 1968.

35: Plato: Timaeus (many translations). Spence, Lewis, *The History of Atlantis* 1926 with many reprints . For a general essay, with substantial references, see: http://en.wikipedia.org/wiki/Atlantis. Of further interest may be MacClean, Ernest G, *The Pythagorean Plato*, Nicholas-Hays,1984

36: The Complete Merlin Tarot, Stewart, R.J. Thorsons, 1992.

37: A short summary with references can be found at: http://en.wikipedia.org/wiki/Theurgy.

38: A short summary with references can be found at: http://en.wikipedia.org/wiki/Triplicity